Emancipatory Perspectives on Madness

This collection offers a diverse range of perspectives that seek to find meaning in madness. Mainstream biomedical approaches tend to interpret experiences commonly labelled "psychotic" as being indicative of a biological illness that can best be ameliorated with prescription drugs. In seeking to counter this perspective, psychosocial outlooks commonly focus on the role of trauma and environmental stress. Although an appreciation for the role of trauma has been critical in expanding the ways in which we view madness, an emphasis of this kind may nevertheless continue to perpetuate a subtle form of reductivism—madness continues to be understood as the product of a deficit. In seeking to move beyond causal-reductivism, this book explores a variety of perspectives on the question of finding inherent meaning in madness and extreme states.

Contributors to this book are distinguished writers and researchers from a variety of international and interdisciplinary perspectives. Topics span the fields of depth psychology and psychoanalysis, creativity, Indigenous and postcolonial approaches, neurodiversity, mad studies, and mysticism and spirituality.

This collection will be of interest to mental health professionals, students and scholars of the humanities and social sciences, and people with lived experience of madness and extreme states. Readers will come away with an appreciation of the more generative aspects of madness, and a recognition that these experiences may be important for both personal and collective healing.

Marie Brown, PhD, is a clinical psychologist, adjunct professor in the Department of Clinical Psychology at Long Island University Brooklyn, and a co-founder of Hearing Voices Network NYC. She is the co-editor (with Marilyn Charles) of *Women and Psychosis: Multidisciplinary Perspectives* and *Women and the Psychosocial Construction of Madness*.

Robin S. Brown, PhD, is a psychoanalyst in private practice and a member of adjunct faculty for the Counseling and Clinical Psychology Department at Teachers College, Columbia University. His first book, *Psychoanalysis Beyond the End of Metaphysics: Thinking Towards the Post-Relational*, won the American Board and Academy of Psychoanalysis Book Prize. This was followed by an edited collection, *Re-Encountering Jung: Analytical Psychology and Contemporary Psychoanalysis*. His most recent publication is *Groundwork for a Transpersonal Psychoanalysis: Spirituality, Relationship, and Participation*.

Emancipatory Perspectives on Madness

Psychological, Social, and Spiritual Dimensions

Edited by Marie Brown & Robin S. Brown

Routledge
Taylor & Francis Group

LONDON AND NEW YORK

First published 2021
by Routledge
2 Park Square, Milton Park, Abingdon, Oxon OX14 4RN

and by Routledge
52 Vanderbilt Avenue, New York, NY 10017

Routledge is an imprint of the Taylor & Francis Group, an informa business

British Library Cataloguing-in-Publication Data
A catalogue record for this book is available from the British Library

Library of Congress Cataloging-in-Publication Data
Names: Brown, Marie, 1981– editor. | Brown, Robin S., editor.
Title: Emancipatory perspectives on madness : psychoanalytic,
    social, and spiritual dimensions / edited by Marie Brown &
    Robin S. Brown.
Description: Abingdon, Oxon ; New York, NY : Routledge, 2021. |
    Includes bibliographical references and index.
Identifiers: LCCN 2020034057 (print) | LCCN 2020034058
    (ebook) | ISBN 9780367360153 (hardback) | ISBN
    9780367360160 (paperback) | ISBN 9780429343261 (ebook)
Subjects: LCSH: Mental illness—Philosophy.
Classification: LCC RC437.5 .E46 2021 (print) | LCC RC437.5
    (ebook) | DDC 616.89001—dc23
LC record available at https://lccn.loc.gov/2020034057
LC ebook record available at https://lccn.loc.gov/2020034058

ISBN: 978-0-367-36015-3 (hbk)
ISBN: 978-0-367-36016-0 (pbk)
ISBN: 978-0-429-34326-1 (ebk)

Typeset in Times New Roman
by Apex CoVantage, LLC

Contents

Contributors

Marilyn Charles, PhD, is a psychologist and psychoanalyst at the Austen Riggs Center in Stockbridge, MA, affiliated with Harvard University, University of Monterrey (UDEM), Boston Graduate School of Psychoanalysis, and Chicago Center for Psychoanalysis. As past president of APA Division 39, she promotes psychodynamic training, community involvement, outreach, and research. She has authored and edited numerous books. Her interests include creativity, psychosis, resilience, and the intergenerational transmission of trauma.

Françoise Davoine, PhD, worked for thirty years as a psychoanalyst in public psychiatric hospitals in France, as an external consultant and is currently in private practice. She was a Professor at the Centre for the Study of Social Movements, École des Hautes Études en Sciences Sociales (EHESS) in Paris, where she and Jean-Max Gaudillière conducted a weekly seminar on "Madness and the Social Link." She is the author of many articles and books, including *La Folie Wittgenstein, Mother Folly*, and *History Beyond Trauma* (with Jean-Max Gaudillière).

Michael Eigen, PhD, is a psychologist and psychoanalyst. He is author of many books and papers, including *The Psychotic Core, The Sensitive Self, Flames from the Unconscious: Trauma, Madness and Faith*, and *The Challenge of Being Human*. He is a senior member of the National Psychological Association for Psychoanalysis and adjunct faculty for the New York University Postdoctoral Program in Psychotherapy and Psychoanalysis. He teaches a weekly private seminar ongoing over forty years.

John Gale is a philosopher and psychotherapist, and was formerly a Benedictine monk. He was a director of a number of organizations in the field of therapeutic communities and was a board member of The International Society for Psychological and Social Approaches to Psychosis UK. He is the author of many scholarly articles at the interface of philosophy, psychoanalysis, and spirituality, and co-edited *Insanity and Divinity: Studies in Psychosis and Spirituality* and *Therapeutic Communities for Psychosis: History, Philosophy, and Clinical Practice*.

Derek Hook, PhD, is an associate professor of psychology at Duquesne University in Pittsburgh, as well as an extraordinary professor in psychology at the University of Pretoria, South Africa. He is author of *6 Moments in Lacan*, *A Critical Psychology of the Postcolonial*, and, with Calum Neill, co-editor of the Palgrave Lacan Series.

Rachel Jane Liebert, PhD, collaborates with decolonizing and feminist scholarship, art and activism to trace the circulation of psy within coloniality and experiment with participatory and more-than-human alternatives. Her 2019 book, *Psycurity: Colonialism, Paranoia and the War on Imagination*, became a performative examination of otherworldly potential within White supremacy; her current project explores embodied, inspirited praxes for engaging colonizer ancestors and doing whiteness differently. A Fulbright and Bright Futures alum, Rachel won the 2016 International Association of Qualitative Inquiry award for her "outstanding" experimentation with method. She is a Senior Lecturer in Psychology at UEL and holds a doctorate from CUNY.

Tim Read, MD, is a consultant psychiatrist who worked for twenty years at the Royal London Hospital, UK. He holds degrees in neuroscience and in medicine, and has also completed trainings in psychoanalytical and transpersonal psychotherapy. He is the author of *Walking Shadows: Archetype and Psyche in Crisis and Growth*.

Ronald Schenk, PhD, is a Jungian analyst practicing in Dallas and Houston. He is a member of the Inter-Regional Society of Jungian Analysts, having served in many administrative positions including president. He has worked on a Navajo Reservation and has created a presentational mode of lecture, song, art, dance, and poetry based on Navajo ceremony. His books include *The Soul of Beauty; Dark Night: Imagination in Everyday Life; The Sunken Quest, the Wasted Fisher, the Pregnant Fish: Essays on a Post-Modern Depth Psychology; and* the most recent, *American Soul: A Cultural Narrative*.

Introduction

What are emancipatory perspectives on madness, and why do they matter?

Marie Brown

The central purpose of this volume is to explore madness from an emancipatory framework. In the most basic sense of the term, to emancipate means "to set free" or "to liberate." When a person is emancipated, they are freed from restraint and control. This may include control at the hands of others (such as in the case of slavery) or control by the power of ideas (such as normative socio-cultural beliefs and customs). In contemporary Euro-American Western culture, the experience of madness is often antithetical to emancipation – hearing voices, alternative states of consciousness, and confusing or "bizarre" behaviors are often *cause* for incarceration, control, and restraint, thereby limiting one's personal freedom. In an essay on forced psychiatric medication and hospitalization, Canadian author Erin Soros (2019) describes the process of being turned from a person into a thing:

> A woman injected the drug deep into my flesh – my bottom bare while my mind braced itself for resistant intelligence to disappear into oblivion. If this encounter had taken place outside of a psychiatric ward, if I were physically assaulted and then penetrated while being held down by multiple men on the street or in any other public or even private place, I would be able to press charges or at least to speak of the crime. But what if the ordeal is sanctioned by the very justice system to which I might turn? What if the police were the ones to deliver me to my treatment?
>
> (p. 117)

A person deemed "mad" is often subject to control by normative ideas regarding "good functioning" and what it means to have a "psychiatric illness." Diagnoses such as schizophrenia or schizoaffective disorder can sound like a life sentence of disability and suffering. These ideas can be so powerfully controlling that they have the potential to rob individuals of their very sense of personhood. In her essay "Recovery and the Conspiracy of Hope," psychiatric survivor and clinical psychologist Pat Deegan (1992) describes the way in which the process of hospitalization and diagnosis can seep into a person's experience of themselves, leading to a profound sense of despair:

> Something way down deep began to break. Slowly the messages of hope-lessness and stigma which so permeated the places we received treat-ment, began to sink in. We slowly began to believe what was being said about us.
>
> (p. 4)

In addition, the phenomenology of madness itself can be experienced as pro-foundly intrusive and restrictive – the feeling that others can hear your private thoughts, or that disembodied voices can control your mind or body, or that people have put cameras inside your home – all can lead to a sense of being controlled by people or things outside of oneself. Sometimes, these experiences can be so terrifying that they lead to a shrinking of one's world, withdrawal from friends or family, an attempt at coping through self-imposed isolation. Sometimes they can lead to a form of mental rigidity or lockdown, this further narrowing one's ability to engage meaningfully with the world:

> While growing up, intrusive thoughts caused a lot of fear and they were sometimes accompanied by impulses which I sometimes couldn't filter. When these thoughts became actions, it usually never resulted in any-thing good. During the outset of my first episode, my lack of control over my impulses was something I sought to control through condition-ing my mind to think in certain ways. I weeded out any and every influ-ence in my life which I felt could create detrimental intrusive thoughts such as TV, movies, most types of music, and I sought isolation to try liberating my mind from anything violent, sexual, or even the slightest bit unscrupulous.
>
> (Anonymous, 2019, p. 3)

To deny these kinds of experiences would be to deny the reality that madness is, for many people, an experience of disenfranchisement. Indeed, attempts to re-imagine madness are often met with criticisms of *romanticizing*, a term that implies making something more appealing than it actually is. For example, R.D. Laing has often been criticized along these lines for interpreting schizo-phrenia as a journey of psychological exploration (Miller, 2009). However, to avoid discussion of the more generative, creative, or liberating aspects of madness in fear of romanticizing can be harmfully reductive. Unger (2019) uses the rational emotive behavior therapy (REBT) term "awfulizing" to dis-cuss the opposite pole of romanticizing, suggesting that not engaging with spiritual/generative/creative conceptualizations of psychosis can lead to an overemphasis on the negative. REBT has long noted that "awfulizing" often causes one to ascribe to the belief that something "absolutely should or must not exist because you find it very bad" (Waltman & Palermo, 2019, p. 45). This type of rhetoric can then lead to increased suffering, as people with psychosis may then struggle to rid themselves of nonvolitional experiences. Societally, awfulizing may promote a particularly damaging form of sanist discourse, which at its most extreme end can appear akin to eugenics, and in its milder forms becomes a rationale for discrimination, incarceration, and the policing of mad persons.

Alternative perspectives on madness, seeking to counter dominant biological or illness narratives, often reconceptualize psychosis as a reaction to trauma and environmental stress. This reconceptualization has been critical in expanding the ways that we think about psychosis, transforming madness from an aberrant sickness to a normative response to horrifying circumstances. However, this way of viewing madness can also perpetuate a subtle form of reductivism. Although no longer an illness, madness is still seen as the product of a deficit or injury. This is reflected in developmental models of madness that view psychosis as a form of being stuck within "primitive" or "infantile" modes of being, this having been brought about by early trauma. It is in this way that theories that seek to be liberating can inadvertently find themselves recapitulating harmful messages of brokenness; messages which can, as Deegan (1992) writes, "sink in" permeating one's mental landscape.

What makes a theory emancipatory?

When a theory is emancipatory, it offers the possibility to liberate a person from personal or societal oppression. In *Writings for a Liberation Psychology*, Martín-Baró (1996) discusses several problematic assumptions of Euro-American psychology that limit its capacity to be liberatory. Most significant for the purposes of the present volume are: positivism, individualism, and ahistoricism. Although Martín-Baró discusses these assumptions within the specific context of Latin American psychology, what he suggests is directly relevant to the question of emancipatory theorizing on madness. His work can be used to emphasize what is limiting, restrictive, and/or confining about mainstream psychiatric/psychological frameworks, and how these assumptions might be subverted by the development of an emancipatory epistemology.

Martín-Baró (1996) first suggests that positivism, or the overreliance on a scientific framework, is unhelpfully restrictive. Positivism disregards any phenomenon that cannot be quantified, measured, or interpreted through logic and reason. Martín-Baró states, "Dividing things up in this way, positivism becomes blind to the most important meanings of human existence" (p. 21). Within the context of madness, the mainstream adoption of positivist assumption has led to an emphasis on illness, deficit, and disease; madness is conceptualized as an experience to be eradicated, suppressed, controlled, and avoided. Arguably, it can be understood that a direct effect of the dominance of positivism has led to the disenfranchisement of mad people as is described by Deegan (1992) and Soros (2019). Sascha Altman DuBrul, co-founder of the radical mental health collective The Icarus Project, describes:

> I've come to believe that somehow, I, like a bunch of the other people who have gravitated to The Icarus Project, have the ability to cross back and forth between different "realms" of reality that most people do not have access to and usually don't even know exist . . . I also believe really strongly that if I, and the other people around me, had different language to talk about what I was going through back then – possibility a language of "spirits" and "possession" – that I never would have gotten locked up in the psych hospital and stuck on all those drugs in the first place.
>
> (Farber, 2012, p. 216)

In the 1800s, Daniel Paul Schreber wrote his book, *Memoirs of My Nervous Illness* for similar reasons. He describes the dual purpose of his book to be both a theological text on the nature of God, in addition to a meditation on the question: "*In what circumstance can a person deemed insane be detained in an asylum against his declared will?*" (Schreber, 1955, p. 313, italics in original). Schreber considered personal freedom inherently linked with the notion of madness-as-divine-communication.

In contrast to positivism, knowledge derived from lived experience often views madness as potentially generative, recognizing that these experiences have their own value. Within the lived-experience paradigm, theories on madness have led to a form of self-emancipation – a freeing of oneself and one's community from the pessimism of mainstream positivistic models. For example, within some lived-experience discourse, there is a re-framing of experiences commonly called mental illness as "mad" or "dangerous gifts," often connected to creativity or particular sensitivities. The concept of "neurodiversity" similarly sees experiences that are commonly called mental *illness* as more appropriately an experience of mental *difference*. Similarly, within theological and spiritual perspectives, madness has often been seen as divine – a direct experience of communion with God.

Martín-Baró (1996) sees another problematic assumption of Euro-American psychology to be *individualism* – a theoretical stance which views all psychological experiences to be of a solely personal nature. His argument is that individualism obfuscates the role of structural factors (such as inequalities and oppression) in the development of psychological distress, turning all problems into "personal problems" (p. 22). Although this is certainly true, and highly relevant to understanding psychosis which disproportionately affects the marginalized, this critique can be extended even further. Individualism also removes the ability to understand madness as holding importance, meaning, or value for the collective. Gregory Bateson's celebrated question highlights this idea:

> What pattern connects the crab to the lobster and the orchid to the primrose and all the four of them to me? And me to you? And all six of us to the amoeba in one direction and to the back-ward schizophrenic in another?
>
> (1979, p. 8)

Theories that have a collectivistic outlook are emancipatory, in that madness is "freed" from the entrapment of being an individual, bodily "problem" into an experience that is connected with the wider humanity. That is, emancipatory epistemologies view madness as relevant not only for an individual's personal experience (e.g. their emotional or spiritual development), but also as inextricably tied to the healing or lives of others, inclusive of their family, community, or greater world. Transpersonal psychiatrist John E. Nelson, states:

> The heart of the psychotic person lies within our own heart; his or her mind is in our mind. Even to pretend competence in meeting such an individual, we must seek within ourselves the wellsprings of all human thought and action. We must learn through fastidious exploration of our deepest selves that every thought, every act ever committed, no matter how hideous or exalted, lies within our own capability. Once we feel this through and through, and also lovingly accept it about ourselves, we will be ready for the encounter with the source of our own madness and that of those we seek to heal. The mad can be our teachers.
>
> (p. 418)

Martín-Baró sees *ahistoricism* as the most problematic assumption of Euro-American psychology. Ahistoricism is the tendency to view all human experience as universally given, existing in the same way across time, history, culture, family, and place. Contemporary biomedical models of madness are quintessential of ahistoricism, contextualizing all behaviors, thoughts and emotions as rooted in the body/brain. A person experiencing voices and visions in the mountains of Peru has the same illness as the person experiencing voices and visions in Idaho, USA. Likewise, ahistoricism disregards the ever-shifting societal conceptualizations of madness across time, often reconfiguring history to be the story of a linear development of scientific progress toward the discovery of brain illnesses. In contrast, emancipatory frameworks use the history of madness to tell a different story, often times bringing past societal conceptualizations into the foreground to be reconsidered. For example, Leslie (2000), in reflecting on the history of madness from the Middle Ages onward, states:

> One thing is certain, madness has a history. Its history inflects in tandem with the needs of the powerful. Madness is the rulebook's cracked mirror.

Sometimes madness has an affinity with freedom, with rejection of the norms of society, its constrictions and codes of conduct. . . . The mad must still insist on that freedom, and find ways of grabbing it.

(p. 82)

Emancipatory epistemologies also engage with non-Western perspectives, recognizing that experiences that fall under the umbrella of "psychosis" in the United States can mean something very different in another context. The synopsis for the film *CRAZYWISE*, directed by Phil Borges, reads:

CRAZYWISE doesn't aim to over-romanticize indigenous wisdom, or completely condemn Western treatment. Not every indigenous person who has a crisis becomes a shaman. And many individuals benefit from Western medications. However, indigenous peoples' acceptance of non-ordinary states of consciousness, along with rituals and metaphors that form deep connections to nature, to each other, and to ancestors, is something we can learn from. CRAZYWISE adds a voice to the growing conversation that believes a psychological crisis can be an opportunity for growth and potentially transformational, not a disease with no cure.

(Crazywise LLC, n.d.)

At the heart of the emancipatory theorizing with which this book is concerned is a commitment to understanding the historical and cultural conceptualizations of madness that have been suppressed or squelched by oppressive sociopolitical, economic, and/or ideological systems. Engaging with these diverse perspectives is important for the re-imagining of what it means to hear voices, see visions, and experiences alternate states of consciousness.

Emancipatory frameworks and personal wellness

If madness is relegated only to the realms of psychiatric illness or psychological suffering, opportunities for self-determined meaning-making are truncated. Lewis (2017) states that allowing for diverse, celebratory, and spiritual interpretations of mental difference is not just a question of epistemology and ontology; it is also a deeply ethical question. Drawing on Foucault, he considers that an ethical imperative of knowledge-creation is to help inform people in making narrative choices about how they understand their experiences. This ability to "story" one's own life has long been a central tenant of the Mad Pride, psychiatric survivor/ex-patient, and radical mental health movements. In *Navigating the Space Between Brilliance and Madness*, The Icarus Project organizers describe such an ethos:

The Icarus Project envisions a new culture and language that resonates with our actual experiences of "mental illness" rather than trying to fit our lives into a conventional framework. We believe we have a dangerous gift to be cultivated and taken care of, rather than a disease or disorder to be "cured" or "eliminated."

(2007, p. 1)

Writers within these forms of discourse (e.g., Mad Studies) often highlight the way in which the pharmaceutical industry, with its vast political and economic power, fuels reductive one-sided narratives about mental illness that permeate Western culture, leaving little room for other approaches (Busfield, 2015). The ability to re-story one's own life, therefore, becomes a political imperative for those who have often felt pushed into adopting medicalized frameworks for self-understanding.

Even within the more mainstream consumer/recovery movement, there is an emphasis on autonomy, choice, and finding one's own path toward recovery. For example, the US Substance Abuse and Mental Health Services Administration [SAMHSA] (2012), defines some of the core components of mental health recovery to include the themes of strength, self-direction, empowerment, holism, and hopefulness. This is intimately tied to one's own personal understanding of their experiences. For example, Kay Redfield Jamison (1996), although using a traditional biomedical framework, simultaneously explores a more creative approach to manic-depression: "is there something about the experience of prolonged periods of melancholia – broken at times by episodes of manic intensity and expansiveness – that leads to a different kind of insight, compassion, and expression of the human condition?" (p. 102). Inclusion of these aspects are important, as approaches which emphasize illness at the expense of deeper meaning can lead to hopelessness. A well-known example from the research literature is the "paradox of insight," whereby individuals who ascribe to a disease conceptualization of their experiences have higher rates of demoralization, depression, and lower quality of life than those who "lack insight" (Lysaker et al., 2018). Similarly, there is the finding that people who recover from schizophrenia are those that are able to dis-identify with "being sick" (Davidson, 2020). Noncausal narratives that emphasize creativity, spirituality, or personal renewal may therefore bring about a sense of possibility, directly impacting the lives of people by connecting them to alternative ways of viewing their experiences.

Emancipatory frameworks and cultural pluralism

Emancipatory frameworks are essential for a commitment to cultural pluralism, multiculturalism, and decolonization. Historicism, as a core feature of emancipatory epistemology, suggests that there are multiple ways of viewing experience, with contemporary Western Euro-American psychiatry being only one of them. In fact, it is impossible to practice within a multicultural framework while simultaneously relying only on positivistic, individualistic, and ahistorical ways of knowing. Although generative or spiritual frameworks for madness are often criticized for romanticizing mental illness, there are many cultures and communities that view alternative states of consciousness from these perspectives. Therefore, criticisms of this kind can betray an implicit form of colonial violence. For example, the windigo is a malevolent spirit that many North American Indigenous people view as capable of inhabiting a person, causing them to become dispossessed, leading to an experience of "windigo psychosis." Indigenous people view this as a spiritual issue or influence and not as a medical illness. Using psychiatric diagnoses or biomedical frameworks to understand this experience could have a negative impact on identity development in Indigenous people, mimicking the loss of cultural identity that occurs through colonization (Linklater, 2014).

The necessity for this commitment to multiculturalism grows ever more apparent with the findings of the World Health Organization (WHO), which demonstrated that disability rates associated with schizophrenia vary according to place, as people in Europe and North America experiencing consistently higher rates of disability than people in India, Africa, and Latin America (Barbato, WHO Nations for Mental Health Initiative, & World Health Organization, 1997). This finding has led many to believe that cultural context has a great deal to do with the expression and outcomes of "schizophrenia." For example, it has been suggested that in India, hallucinations may be closer to common religious practices than in North America, marking these types of experiences as more normative (Luhrmann, 2007). In Ghana, individuals experiencing hallucinations and delusions who believe they are suffering from witchcraft sometimes rapidly improve after visiting a local shrine, a finding congruent with the fact that fewer people develop chronic schizophrenia in non-Western settings (Droney, 2016). This concept regarding culture and madness was also suggested in the writings of anti-colonialist psychiatrist Frantz Fanon during the 1950s. In reflecting on the Maghrebi Muslims in Algeria, Fanon and Sanchez (1956) discuss how people experiencing madness within that community were never socially excluded as was typical in Western culture, due to the belief that the person's behavior was caused by wicked genies rather than an illness. Fanon and Sanchez state that individuals experiencing madness in Algeria were sometimes the saint-like object of veneration by the collective, or were alternatively respected more simply as a human being struggling with powerful spirits. Fanon and Sanchez outline this response in contrast to Western culture, which they describe as adopting an illness framework while nonetheless understanding the mad individual as agentic in their "bizarre" or "odd" behaviors. Fanon and Sanchez use this example to question the ethics of European mental healthcare in the practice of isolating people from the community of others.

In discussing the ever-growing influence of Western psychiatric ideology across the globe, Ethan Watters (2010) author of *Crazy Like Us: The Globalization of the American Psyche*, states, "We should worry about this loss of diversity in the world's differing conceptions and treatments of mental illness is exactly the same way we worry about the loss of biological diversity in nature" (p. 7). To deny alternative ways of viewing madness would be to contribute to a problematic homogenizing of global cultures. Much like the ecological benefits of diversity in the world of plants and animals, diversity in the world of ideas and culture can similarly be understood as a marker of health. Emancipatory perspectives may therefore play a role in ensuring the continued complexity and well-being of our human world.

Emancipatory frameworks and collective transformation

On the societal or collective level, emancipatory perspectives have the potential to change the mental healthcare system, paving the way for more humane approaches. Those figures who have tended to most emphasize a nonpositivistic stance regarding madness have also tended to create less restrictive environments for treatment. For example, R.D. Laing's emphasis on psychosis as a potentially transformative event led to the establishment of Kingsley Hall, a place for people with psychosis to go through the experience without locked doors. Similarly, John Weir Perry's belief in the spiritual foundation of psychosis led to the creation of Diabasis, a residential facility for young adults that limited the use of medication. This pattern can also be seen cross-culturally. For example, a Turkish study found that people who believed psychosis was an illness of the brain were more in favor of approaches which emphasized restrictive living than were people who believed in *ruhsal hastagi*, or the idea that psychosis is an issue of the spirit or inner self (Watters, 2010). This relationship between emancipatory perspectives on madness and transformation of the mental health system is nowhere more apparent than in the name of the human rights organization Mind Freedom International, where the ability to have freedom of thought about one's own experiences and psyche is inextricably linked to re-imagining a humane, noncoercive, nonviolent, mental health care system.

Regardless of transformations in the mental health care system, emancipatory perspectives also underscore the value of madness for the collective on an even broader level. Certain theorists have conceptualized madness as an agent of change within problematic familial patterns. Haley (1997), for example, views madness as at first providing a regulatory, stabilizing function for families, which can then bring about needed re-organization following a crisis. Indeed, within the family therapy tradition, there is a long-established idea that the person at the center of concern is bringing the family into closer contact with an experience that is needed for healing. Bowen (1966) states: "The family is a system in that a change in one part of the system is followed by compensatory change in other parts of the system" (p. 351). A person experiencing recovery/renewal through an experience of madness then triggers a change in another family member, and then another, eventually leading to a transformation within the family system as a whole. This change or transformation can be seen as benefiting the immediate family, but may also reflect a form of healing from trauma within past generations. Importantly, these types of views do not blame family members as casual factors to an individual's madness, but instead emphasize the importance of interconnectedness.

Hoffman (1981) extends these concepts outside of the family sphere toward the greater world. She describes the process of morphogenesis, whereby a positive feedback loop works to amplify deviation, which then allows for needed mutation or transformation in order for the collective to adjust to a changed environment. She discusses the ways in which chaos, rather than being something undesirable, can have a positive value in the face of "negentropy," or too much structure, a condition which is ultimately detrimental due to the extreme constriction it places upon people. Her words on the potential for chaos to promote newness or stagnation can easily be applied to the value of madness:

> the growth of monopolies might lead to such total inequity that social revolution would result, *or* it could inspire a movement toward antitrust legislation. The death of a religious or political heretic might reinforce the system he repudiated, or his martyrdom might lead to a revision of the entire social order. The death or suicide of a family member might close off possibilities for change in the family, or it might release unexpected potential for growth.
>
> (p. 52, italics in original)

Many people have described hearing voices, seeing visions, or experiencing alternative states of consciousness as "the canary in the coalmine" – experiences that reveal a fault within existing social structures that needs to be examined. For example, The Mindful Occupation Collective (2019) states,

> a lot of us have visions about how things could be different, why they need to be different, and it's painful to keep them silent. Sometimes we get called sick and sometimes we get called sacred, but no matter how they name us, we are a vital part of making this planet whole.
>
> (p. 145)

Returning to a cross-cultural framework, experiences that in the West may be called "madness," are sometimes implicated in the communal processing of trauma. For example, de Jong and Reis (2013) studying a group of Balanta women in Guinea-Bissau observed the way in which the women's distress, inclusive of spirit possession or "dissociation," can be understood as a "symbolic language addressing politically dangerous truths," lending itself to the possibility for collective healing through a "pathway to mitigate the consequences of protracted and widespread political violence" (p. 644). These ways of viewing madness are more than just postmodern attempts at "re-storying" individual experience – madness is respected for the inherent value it holds in transforming others.

Conclusion

The present volume brings together many different perspectives, all with an emancipatory orientation toward the question of madness. Whether psychodynamic, transpersonal, spiritual/ mystical, or decolonial, each author endeavors to bring about a sense of possibility and wonder – two qualities often trapped or obfuscated under the heavy weight of illness narratives. Bateson (1979) contrasts two conceptions of the world, the *pleroma* and the *creatura*, with the *pleroma* being descriptive of the nonliving world of "billiard-ball cause-and-effect," and the *creatura* as the living world, of differences and distinctions, inherently interconnected. It is our hope, in editing this book, to help foster a conversation that would move beyond "nonliving" perspectives on madness.

Importantly, emancipatory perspectives on madness have the potential to reveal to us a world imbued with meaning, purpose, and interconnection. Bateson (1979) believed that the recognition of a fundamental unity – of people, mind, and the biosphere – is essential for the survival of human life on the planet. This mode of thinking is in sharp distinction to the disenchantment of contemporary Western culture, which views the world as fragmented and disconnected. From this perspective, theorizing on madness from an emancipatory perspective matters because the way in which we understand ourselves and the mental experiences of others parallels the conclusions we draw about the world as a whole. If we view madness as a process that – with patience and care – can bring about regeneration, renewal, and growth, we may in turn meet the struggles of the world's stage with the same faith that within the turmoil, there is a striving toward something meaningful.

References

Anonymous. (2019). Intrusive thoughts, impulses, and schizoaffective disorder. *Schizophrenia Bulletin, 45*(1), 3–4.

Barbato, A., WHO Nations for Mental Health Initiative, & World Health Organization. (1997). *Schizophrenia and public health* (No. WHO/MSA/NAM/97.6). World Health Organization. https://apps.who.int/iris/handle/10665/63837.

Bateson, G. (1979). *Mind and nature: A necessary unity*. New York: Bantam Books.

Bowen, M. (1966). The use of family theory in clinical practice. *Comprehensive Psychiatry, 7*(5), 345–374.

Busfield, J. (2015). The pharmaceutical industry and mental disorder. In S. Coles, S. Keenan, & B. Diamond (Eds.), *Madness contested: Power and practice*. Ross-On-Wye, UK: PCCS Books Ltd.

Crazywise LLC. (n.d.). *CRAZYWISE synopsis*. https://crazywisefilm.com/crazywise-synopsis/.

Davidson, L. (2020). Recovering a sense of self in schizophrenia. *Journal of Personality*, *88*(1), 122–132.

de Jong, J., & Reis, R. (2013). Collective trauma processing: Dissociation as a way of processing postwar traumatic stress in Guinea Bissau. *Transcultural Psychiatry*, *50*(5), 644–661.

Deegan, P. (1992). *Recovery, rehabilitation and the conspiracy of hope*. Lawrence, MA: National Empowerment Center.

Droney, D. (2016). Demonic voices: One man's experience of god, witches, and psychosis in Accra, Ghana. In T. M. Luhrmann & J. Marrow (Eds.), *Our most troubling madness: Case studies in schizophrenia across cultures*. Berkeley: University of California Press.

Fanon, F., & Sanchez, F. (1956). Maghrebi Muslims and their attitude to madness. In F. Fanon (Ed.), *Alienation and freedom*. London, UK: Bloomsbury Publishing.

Farber, S. (2012). *The spiritual gift of madness: The failure of psychiatry and the rise of the mad pride movement*. New York: Simon and Schuster.

Haley, J. (1997). *Leaving home: The therapy of disturbed young people*. Abingdon, UK: Routledge.

Hoffman, L. (1981). *Foundations of family therapy*. New York: Basic Books.

The Icarus Project. (2007). *Navigating the space between brilliance and madness: A readers & roadmap of bipolar worlds [Pamphlet]*. n.p.: Icarus Project.

Jamison, K. R. (1996). *Touch with fire: Manic-depressive illness and the artistic temperament*. New York: Free Press.

Leslie, E. (2000). Mad pride and prejudice. In T. Curtis, R. Dellar, E. Leslie & B. Watson (Eds.), *Mad pride: A celebration of mad culture*. London, UK: Spare Change Books.

Lewis, B. (2017). A deep ethics for mental difference and disability: The 'case' of Vincent van Gogh. *Medical Humanities*, *43*, 172–176.

Linklater, R. (2014). *Decolonizing trauma work: Indigenous stories and strategies*. Novia Scotia, Canada: Fernwood Publishing.

Luhrmann, T. M. (2007). Social defeat and the culture of chronicity: Or, why schizophrenia does so well over there and so badly here. *Culture, Medicine and Psychiatry*, *31*(2), 135–172.

Lysaker, P. H., Pattison, M. L., Leonhardt, B. L., Phelps, S., & Vohs, J. L. (2018). Insight in schizophrenia spectrum disorders: Relationship with behavior, mood and perceived quality of life, underlying causes and emerging treatments. *World Psychiatry*, *17*(1), 12–23.

Martín-Baró, I. (1996). *Writings for a liberation psychology*. Cambridge, MA: Harvard University Press.

Miller, G. (2009). R. D. Laing and theology: The influence of Christian existentialism on the divided self. *History of the Human Sciences*, *22*(2), 1–21.

Mindful Occupation Collective. (2019). What is radical mental health? In L. D. Green & K. Ubozoh (Eds.), *We've been too patient: Voices from radical health*. Berkeley, CA: North Atlantic Books.

Nelson, J. E. (1990). *Healing the split: A new understanding of the crisis and treatment of the mentally ill*. New York: Jeremy P. Tarcher, Inc.

Schreber, D. P. (1955). *Memoirs of my nervous illness*. New York: New York Review of Books Classics.

Soros, E. (2019). I call this institutionalized rape. In M. C. Brown & M. Charles (Eds.), *Women and the psychosocial construction of madness*. Lanham, MD: Lexington Books.

Substance Abuse and Mental Health Services Administration [SAMHSA]. (2012). *SAMHSA's working definition of recovery [Brochure]*. Rockville, MD. http://store.samhsa.gov/shin/.

Unger, R. (2019, May 14). Recovery vs mad pride: Exploring the contradictions. In *Recovery from "Schizophrenia" and other "Psychotic Disorders" [BLOG]*. Eugene: Newstex.

Waltman, S. H., & Palermo, A. (2019). Theoretical overlap and distinction between rational emotive behavior therapy's awfulizing and cognitive therapy's catastrophizing. *Mental Health Review Journal, 24*(1), 44–50.

Watters, E. (2010). *Crazy like us: The globalization of the American psyche*. New York: Free Press.

Chapter 1

On the potential limits of trauma theory as an emancipatory discourse[1]

Robin S. Brown

ABSTRACT: This chapter suggests that a clinical reliance on causal-reductive thinking further accentuates the sense of alienation experienced by people under-going psychosis, and that trauma-based approaches to psychosis should therefore be adopted with care. Arguing against an emphasis on notions of developmental deficit, the author explores how psychoanalytic thinking might question some of the paradigmatic assumptions of clinical psychology.

KEYWORDS: psychoanalysis, psychosis, spirituality, teleology, trauma

Constrictive views of psychosis have the effect of further isolating the afflicted. With this in mind, in so far as clinicians cannot avoid betraying their own assumptions (whether explicitly formulated as "theoretical" or otherwise), a good theory helps the clinician to assume a more self-reflexive position and facilitates communication. Psychoanalytic thinking has sought to find ways of working with the clinician's assumptions, either (from a classical perspective) to minimize interference with the patient's process or (from a more relational perspective) so that the influence of the clinician's personality might have a positive impact on the therapeutic process. The shift from one-person to two-person models of practice has often been taken to signify a less dogmatic approach to theory, wherein the clinician's theoretical supports should not occlude the lived experience of the patient. However, in so far as approaches of this kind proceed on the basis of ideas pertaining to the causative nature of human relationships, more can yet be done in challenging paradigmatic assumptions.

Teleology in psychoanalysis

Throughout the history of psychoanalysis, the scientifically respectable ambience of a causal-reductive approach to the psyche has always been muddied with elements of teleology. A teleological approach would seek to understand a certain phenomenon not in terms of its material causes, but rather with a view to its final purpose or goal. The birth of modern science saw the exclusion of final causes as a subject fit for study, with mechanistic models of understanding being considered a marker of objectivity. Francis Bacon has sometimes been misunderstood to have sought to delegitimate teleology altogether:

> Bacon holds that the existence of teleology in Nature is an obvious fact, and that the investigation of final causes is a perfectly legitimate branch of Natural Philosophy. It has, however, been misplaced; for it belongs to the division of Natural Philosophy which Bacon calls *Metaphysics* and not to that which he calls *Physics*. Bacon's epigram that "the research into Final Causes, like a virgin dedicated to God, is barren and produces nothing" has been taken by careless or biased readers to be a condemnation of such research. It is nothing of the kind. It is simply a statement of the obvious fact that there is no art of Applied Teleology as there is an art of Applied Physics.
>
> (Broad, 1926, para. 8)

In contrast to an approach which would seek to entirely exclude teleology from scientific practice, Immanuel Kant argued that for the sake of scientific advance teleology serves a necessary heuristic purpose. Teleology is positioned by Kant as a regulative principle. In scientific discovery, teleological thinking enables us to achieve a picture of a whole that is not yet known. He considers that cognition relies upon the metaphor of final purpose in order to achieve scientific insight, yet this teleological scaffold must ultimately be discarded if we are to achieve objective scientific knowledge. However, Kant argues that our understanding of living organisms simply cannot be resolved into mechanical terms since the thing that we seek to grasp will always elude our total comprehension. In the *Critique of Judgment*, he considers an organism as both cause and effect of itself.

For early psychoanalysts, particular stress was placed on understanding a person's psychology in terms of early childhood. Freud's notion of "psychic determinism" has often been interpreted along mechanistic lines to mean that the patient's psychological life can be explained in purely causal terms. As Brenner (1955) puts it:

> The sense of this principle is that in the mind, as in physical nature about us, nothing happens by chance, or in a random way. Each psychic event is determined by the ones that precede it. Events in our mental lives that may seem to be random and unrelated to what went on before are only apparently so. In fact, mental phenomena are no more capable of such a lack of causal connection with what preceded them than are physical ones.
>
> (p. 2)

Despite the materialist and deterministic tone of Freud's work, Basch (1978) argues that the strictly causal lines along which Freud's notion of psychic determinism has often been interpreted is a misreading, and that Freud did in fact knowingly seek to allow for some question of intentionality:

> Motivation, purposiveness and goal-directedness are terms that have often been, and still are in many quarters, looked at askance. They suggest that there is an ephemeral cause that beckons from afar and guides behaviour according to some design of its own. Freud was aware of this danger and tried to avoid it by refusing to entertain any notion of purpose or plan that went beyond causality rooted in the findings of physics or chemistry. Freud's models for goal directed action were energy conversion apparatuses analogous to then recently invented machines like the electric lamp, the telegraph and the telephone. . . . A lamp or telephone cannot be said to have a goal; it is the user who has a purpose in mind when he turns it on. For this reason Freud's attempt to design a mental apparatus along the lines of the physics of his day proved to be unsatisfactory. He had to introduce purpose into the simple reflex construct he designed by postulating unobservable homunculi . . . like the unconscious, the instincts, the ego, etc., each having its own aim and struggling for power. The very teleology that Freud sought to avoid by adhering to the thermodynamic laws of natural science was introduced into psychoanalysis by . . . his explanatory models.
>
> (p. 260)

Rather than looking to ascertain how a certain thing came about, the teleological perspective is concerned with goal directedness. Any psychological approach that endorses a basic human tendency toward healing, wholeness, or health can be considered teleological in outlook. Such notions are essential if symptoms are to be respected as having a potential value. Notwithstanding American ego psychology's penchant for pathologizing and authoritarianism, the history of psychoanalysis is in fact rife with teleological concepts. A few examples would include:

- Adler's (1938) emphasis on the source of human motivation lying in the future rather than the past
- Rank's (1936) focus on creativity
- Jung's (1947) psychology of individuation as reflected in the prospective function of the psyche in its movement toward wholeness
- Bion's (1965) notion of a truth drive
- Winnicott's (1971) concept of a true self realized in play and expressive of an inherent tendency toward growth
- Kohut's (1977) self-psychological outlook as reflected in the spontaneously felt need for selfobject experiences
- Loewald's (1980) thinking on sublimation
- Bollas's (2018) notions of personal idiom and destiny drive

Significantly, these ideas tend to moderate the relational emphasis on context and make room for some question of individual purposiveness.

Conceptualizing trauma

Any sense that mental illness might be considered purposive tends to imply what might loosely be termed a *spiritual* orientation toward practice. This naturally rubs up against conventional psychiatric assumption. In so far as spiritual issues are occasionally tolerated within mainstream thinking on psychosis, this is typically framed in terms of how religious or spiritual beliefs might be considered supportive of a patient's well-being (Phillips & Stein, 2007). While there is no doubt value in this approach, a polite engagement of this kind still tends to neglect the more fundamental sense in which the clinician's own spiritual commitments impact treatment. These commitments unavoidably emerge in theorizing about the nature and treatment of madness.

In the extent to which psychological attitudes toward psychosis have come to rely on the empirically verifiable role of trauma (Read, van Os, Morrison, & Ross, 2005), the fashion in which trauma theory is incorporated into clinical theorizing is of central importance. A teleological outlook on trauma tends to get neglected wherever our thinking leans too heavily on normative ideas about human development. Developmental approaches often emphasize a perceived deficit in the patient's early experience leading to modes of functioning that are considered less than optimal. From this perspective, disruptions to good caregiving can be understood as the crux of intergenerational trauma. A few examples:

- Fraiberg, Adelson, and Shapiro (1975) perceive that recovery from the cycle of traumatization is dependent on the child of a traumatized parent refusing to identify with the aggressor. Where such an identification occurs, affect is thought to be split off in the child, only to return as a distortion in subsequent parenting skills.
- Drawing from Stern's (1997) developmental theory, Adelman (1995, p. 363) conceptualizes transmission in terms of a disruption to the organization of the verbal self. For Adelman, trauma is transmitted by way of the relationship between a parent's capacity to modulate their child's affect and the child's resultant capacity to verbalize.
- Bradfield (2011) is explicit when he conceptualizes the attachment relationship as the "location" of the child's traumatic experience. The child's need for containment is thought to elicit fear or rage in the traumatized parent, thus disturbing the attachment bond.

Whether considered in terms of split-off affect, unsymbolized experience, or attachment bonds, the belief subtending these theories is that the interpersonal transmission of trauma is fundamentally concerned with a deficit in the experience of early relationships. It is thus proposed that these deficits might subsequently be ameliorated in the work of therapy. Where there is a focus on trauma as causative of psychological deficits, however, and trauma is treated as the foundation of psychosis, there is a clear risk of conceptualizing psychotic experience merely in terms of an environmental shortfall.

Davoine and Gaudillière (2004) have developed a noteworthy clinical approach that seeks to avoid inadvertently infantilizing their patients. In *History Beyond Trauma*, they offer an unconventional approach to madness that they regard as nonreductive. Eschewing biological reductionism, they follow the notion that psychosis is connected to trauma. However, they expand upon this position by emphasizing the extent to which all trauma ultimately relates to the events of our collective history. Perceiving their patients as researchers, they see the clinician's role not as that of a healer, but rather as an assistant to the work of historical research: "Sometimes a fit of madness tells us more than all the news dispatches about the left-over facts that have no right to existence" (p. xxvii). For Davoine and Gaudillière, to speak of something actively traumatic having been *forgotten* is misleading, in that the trauma cannot properly be said to reside in the past. The place of trauma is inferred by an absence, this being conceivable as a gap in the signifying chain of collective history. Recovery is achieved not by seeking to find containment for the unconscious (as psychoanalytic approaches that emphasize the need of a "strong ego" might assume), or by attempting to unearth something forgotten, but rather by trying to create the possibility of a repression – and hence, the hope of being able to forget. The unsymbolized trauma cannot be said to belong to the past, because it is precisely the existence of the trauma in the present that demands attention.

Accepting the patient's experience requires that the clinician confront a conflict in themselves and move beyond causal thinking. The traumatic event is not yet an event at all, but rather the implication of something not yet nameable. Only at the intersection of shared experiences evoked by the therapeutic dyad can the patient give voice to the unspeakable. For the analyst to play a part in this means allowing the patient to lead – the clinician should view themselves as a co-participant. This entails the clinician divulging experiences of their own emerging relationship to trauma; a gesture that would more usually be considered intrusive, but out of which an alliance is formed enabling the shared process of forging history. Where conventional practice might dissuade an analyst from sharing elements of their own experience with the patient, particularly if the material is emotionally demanding, paying this kind of testimony to trauma is in this context regarded as essential.

By emphasizing the role of collective history, Davoine and Gaudillière offer an example of an approach to trauma that moves beyond interpersonal conceptions of transmission. This is not to the exclusion of the role that interpersonal factors play in giving rise to traumatic experience, but in the extent that we continue to consider these factors a cause, their effect is no longer to be perceived as the kernel of the trauma itself so much as a heightened receptivity to it – the trauma informs the sense of a calling which, in effect, enables the patient to conduct the work of historical research. Patients experiencing psychosis are often tortured by the efforts of others to "explain" psychotic experience causally.[2] For this reason, the only means of making a genuine connection with the patient is by way of coincidence. A clinician may discover, for instance, that the patient's grandfather was critically injured during a battle in which the clinician's own paternal grandfather was also hurt. Coincidences by definition pose a challenge to the logic of causal reasoning and hence provide a nonthreatening means of drawing closer to the patient. The unexpected and sometimes mysterious ways in which the patient's relationship to trauma coincides with that of the clinician is the bond by means of which communication becomes possible.[3]

The role of the individual

For Davoine and Gaudillière, the effort to symbolize the unspeakable is an undertaking to introduce something new into the established order. Where Davoine and Gaudillière speak of breaks in the chain of signification, the transpersonal theorist Michael Washburn (1995) speaks of black holes in psychic space: "interruptions in internal dialogue can occur. And these interruptions are not periods of restful, much less serene, silence; they are rather moments of trancelike blankness, moments during which internal dialogue is extinguished" (p. 188). Davoine and Gaudillière's view suggests that absences of this kind point to traumatic gaps in the collective historical record. Their challenging work might therefore cause us to question the often individualistic basis upon which teleological assumptions come to rest. In particular, the notion in humanistic psychology and the human potential movement that self-realization is the de facto goal of human endeavor (Laszlo, 1996, p. 82) appears less definitive. This position, which stands as one of the foundational assumptions of the transpersonal psychology movement, has in recent years been critiqued as part of Jorge Ferrer's call for a "participatory turn" in transpersonal theorizing. Ferrer (2002) questions the legitimacy of assuming that spiritual transformation is a fundamentally private affair. This needn't imply neglecting the transformative agency of the individual, but it does suggest that it may be shortsighted to conceive of experiences as spiritual only if they can be shown to directly benefit the individual. Davoine and Gaudillière's approach to trauma demonstrates how teleology need not imply self-realization. That which is seeking to find expression is fundamentally a question posed to the collective and not merely to the experience of the individual.[4]

For Davoine and Gaudillière, the person's experience is perceived as a conduit to those gaps in the symbolic order that register the existence of an unsymbolized trauma. In other words, the question of a deficit is no longer imputed to the patient, but rather to the collective, and it is the patient who seeks to ameliorate for this deficit by attending to an absence in the historical record. The dignity thus reserved for the individual in this scheme is in stark contrast to the treatment of intergenerational trauma understood in terms of a correction to the patient's developmental shortcomings realized by way of relationship to the therapist. When evaluating our theoretical tools, the implicit value accorded to the individual needs to be considered paramount if clinicians are to avoid adopting restrictive modes of perceiving their patients. If an assumption is made that the individual is nothing more than a consequence of the material conditions from which he or she arises, then the only way in which to understand psychosis (or, for that matter, any other psychological struggle) is in terms of genetics or immediate social and environmental influences. By contrast, if the individual is posited to be influenced in some degree by factors that transcend immediate material causes, then it becomes conceivable that the individual's experience may carry a meaning for the material situation that is not immediately reducible to it.

Although Freud's drive theory is justifiably perceived by many as excessively reductive, his approach nevertheless assigns a certain implicit value to the role of the individual: the drives are thought to be attached to persons; hence, their regulation is essentially an individual problem. Freud's tendency to think in terms of the individual has, for good reason, been questioned since the inception of his work. However, the shift away from drive in favor of more relational models, while freeing psychoanalytic theory from the dogmatism associated with the field's early development, has at times implicitly diminished the role of the individual as a locus of creative agency. For example, the work of Harry Stack Sullivan's (1950) can give the impression that the individual is being portrayed as an illusion consisting of nothing more than the role a person plays in relationship to others. The advantage of such a position in terms of the theorizing of psychosis is clear: by radically questioning the notion of the individual, Sullivan's work calls for a shift in the perception of mental illness from something that exists "in" persons, to something that is enacted between persons. But while this point of view might help emancipate the sufferer from being stigmatized, this perspective also implies that the individual's experience is always reducible to the status quo and as such can never be expected to radically transform it.

If the message of madness is related only to a call for the rearrangement of the environmental situation as it stands – or, even more reductively, as a call for the rearrangement of the internalized environmental conditions of the past – then we are left with an approach that would seek always to understand madness in terms of a set of circumstances that were less than "ideal." It is in questioning this supposed ideal, however, that madness may in fact be most centrally concerned. R.D. Laing (1967), working from a systems perspective influenced by Gregory Bateson, nonetheless seems to perceive the ideological danger that emerges when the individual is reduced to nothing more than their environmental circumstances. Laing writes: "There are men who feel called upon to generate even themselves out of nothing, since their underlying feeling is that they have not been adequately created or have been created only for destruction" (pp. 42–43).

Autopoiesis is a term introduced by Maturana and Varela (1980) to characterize the organization of living systems. It signifies the fashion in which life produces and maintains itself as a process. Organisms are understood in this light as a product of their own production, and it is through this ongoing act of self-production that organisms render themselves distinct within an environment upon which they are nonetheless dependent. The related notion of *enaction* was subsequently introduced to describe a theory by which cognition is understood to arise in dynamic relationship between an autopoietic organism and the environment:

> We propose as a name the term *enactive* to emphasize the growing conviction that cognition is not the representation of a pre-given world by a pre-given mind but is rather the enactment of a world and a mind on the basis of a history of the variety of actions that a being in the world performs.
>
> (Varela, Thompson, & Rosch, 1991, p. 9, italics in original)

With an enactivist perspective, the notion that the whole is more than the sum of its parts can be supplemented with a counter position: that the parts are themselves wholes that are more than the function they play in relationship to that whole of which they can be considered a part. Within the clinical setting, this outlook allows us to conceptualize the relationship between therapist and patient as an autonomous system *and* to consider both participants as autonomous systems in their own right. Of particular significance for a cogent ethical justification for clinical work, such an approach allows for the possibility of personal agency:

> Autopoiesis takes the "self" in self-organization seriously. It establishes agency – and consequently downward causation – as a central property of living systems and requires the framing of living phenomena in final causal, teleological terms, wherein "purposiveness" or "that for the sake of which" provides a key component of scientific explanation. Autopoietic systems construct themselves by generating the very constraints that establish far-from-equilibrium conditions, demonstrating an agency through self-determination.
>
> (Witherington, 2011, p. 80)

In the history of psychology, the substance of the "nature versus nurture" debate has been skewed from the outset in terms of a polarity that normalizes causal-reductive thinking. By considering individual differences as determined (rather than formed) by material causes, the individual's experience is rendered devoid of meaning, with whatever value might be imputed to this experience only being registered in the terms of the system as it stands. Ludwig von Bertalanffy, one of the pioneers of systems theory, was nonetheless acutely aware of what he perceived to be the dangers of assuming a systems standpoint to the detriment of the individual. He considers the emergence of systems thinking to be a profoundly ambivalent phenomenon in the history of ideas, recognizing the dehumanizing propensity that is attendant to it and the fashion in which this tendency tends to reinforce existing social problems:

> Man in the Big System is to be – and to a large extent has become – a moron, buttonpusher or learned idiot, that is, highly trained in some narrow speciali-zation but otherwise a mere part of the machine. This conforms to a well-known systems principle, that of progressive mechanization the individual becoming ever-more a cogwheel dominated by a few privileged leaders, mediocrities and mystifiers who pursue their private interests under a smoke-screen of ideologies.
>
> (1968, p. 10)

In light of such a position, we might reflect upon the political implications of Judith Herman's (1997) notion that recovery from trauma is ultimately dependent on giving up a belief in one's own specialness. There is an implicit sense of the individual's defeat in this claim. This becomes more appreciable when psychosis is regarded not as a meaningless aberration conditioned by less than ideal cir-cumstances in the gene pool and/or childhood environment, but as an unshakable commitment to express a particular message.

Notes

1 Sections of this chapter are revised from a previously published paper titled "An Open-ing: Trauma and Transcendence" (Brown, 2015).
2 As Perry (2005) states: "The more sane-making we become in our good will, the more crazy-making we find ourselves; we entangle ourselves in our own preconceptions, and the patient becomes hopelessly ensnared along with us" (p. 130).
3 While working primarily from a Lacanian basis, the emphasis Davoine and Gaudillière place on coincidence potentially brings their approach into conversation with Jungian psychology. Throughout his work, Jung (1954) maintains that psychic and somatic dis-turbances cannot be understood purely in terms of their etiology: "Besides the cause and the unknown X of the individual's disposition, we must also take into account the teleological aspects of fitness in biology, which in the psychic realm would have to be formulated as *meaning*" (p. 342, italics in original). The problem of ancestral memory is also central to Jung's work – the notion of a "collective" unconscious perhaps being the clearest expression of this. Jung's own sense of meaning, as expressed in the private mythology portrayed in *The Red Book* (2009), seems to have hinged upon the unre-solved questions inherited from foregoing generations: "It seemed [to Jung] that the dead only knew what they knew when they died, hence their tendency to intrude into our lives. In this regard he found the Chinese custom that events should be conveyed to the ancestors to be very significant" (Shamdasani, 2008, p. 19). Jung's (1952) notion of synchronicity still reflects the most significant treatment of the psychological value of acausal coincidences, with the underlying theoretical basis for this notion being funda-mental to the development of his work (see Brown, 2018, 2020). Additionally, the clas-sical Jungian technique of "amplifying" the patient's material by drawing comparisons from myth might be considered in some degree parallel to Davoine and Gaudillière's method of shared historical inquiry. Shamdasani (Hillman & Shamdasani, 2013) sug-gests that Jungian amplification is essentially "storytelling," emphasizing that Jung's use

of mythology allows him to move away from psychodynamics and to do service to the experience of being particularly oneself (p. 89).

4 This has implications for the convention of categorizing different kinds of psychotic experience in terms of their supposed spiritual validity. Stanislav Grof is a prominent spokesperson for the notion that a distinction can be drawn between medical psychosis and spiritual crisis: "mainstream psychiatry and psychology in general make no distinction between mysticism and mental illness" (Grof & Grof, 1989, p. 2). This distinction can be traced at least as far back as Boisen (1936), who in similar fashion seeks to outline a difference between organic psychosis and authentic problems of religious transformation. It is also reflected in the classical Jungian notion that the first half of life should be given over to the development of a robust ego such as to be able to subsequently withstand the initiatory experience of a dark night of the soul, in which context the "pathological" forms of breakdown are thought to be indicative of an unprepared psychic vessel. While the distinction being made certainly seems to speak to a qualitative difference in the experience of psychosis, it is perhaps misleading to suppose that this difference characterizes the extent to which the experience can be considered spiritual.

References

Adelman, A. (1995). Traumatic memory and the intergenerational transmission of holocaust narratives. *Psychoanalytic Study of the Child, 50*, 343–367.

Adler, A. (1938). *Social interest: A challenge to mankind*. Eastford, CT: Martino Fine Books.

Basch, M. F. (1978). Psychic determinism and freedom of will. *The International Review of Psycho-Analysis, 5*, 257–264.

Bion, W. R. (1965). Memory and desire. In *The complete works of W.R. Bion* (Vol. VI, pp. 7–17). London: Karnac Books.

Boisen, A. T. (1936). *The exploration of the inner world*. New York: Harper & Brothers.

Bollas, C. (2018). *Forces of destiny: Psychoanalysis and human idiom*. London & New York: Routledge.

Bradfield, B. (2011). The dissociation of lived experience: A relational psychoanalytic analysis of the intergenerational transmission of trauma. *International Journal of Psychoanalytic Self Psychology, 6*, 531–550.

Brenner, C. (1955). *An elementary textbook of psychoanalysis*. New York: International University Press.

Broad, C. D. (1926). *The philosophy of francis bacon: An address delivered at cambridge on the occasion of the bacon tercentenary*. Cambridge: Cambridge University Press.

Brown, R. S. (2015). An opening: Trauma and transcendence. *Psychosis: Psychological, Social and Integrative Approaches, 7*(1), 72–80.

Brown, R. S. (2018). Imaginal action: Towards a jungian conception of enactment, and an extraverted counterpart to active imagination. *Journal of Analytical Psychology, 63*(2), 186–206.

Brown, R. S. (2020). *Groundwork for a transperonal psychoanalysis: Spirituality, relationship, and participation*. London & New York: Routledge.

Davoine, F., & Gaudillière, J. (2004). *History beyond trauma*. New York: Other Press.

Ferrer, J. N. (2002). *Revisioning transpersonal theory: A participatory vision of human spirituality*. Albany, NY: SUNY Press.

Fraiberg, S., Adelson, E., & Shapiro, V. (1975). Ghosts in the nursery: A psychoanalytic approach to the problems of impaired infant-mother relationships. *Journal of the American Academy of Child Psychiatry*, *14*, 387–421.

Grof, C., & Grof, S. (Eds.). (1989). *Spiritual emergency: When personal transformation becomes a crisis*. New York: Penguin Putnam.

Herman, J. (1997). *Trauma and recovery*. New York: Basic Books.

Hillman, J., & Shamdasani, S. (2013). *Lament of the dead: Psychology after jung's red book*. New York: W. W. Norton & Company.

Jung, C. G. (1947). On the nature of the psyche. In *Collected works* (Vol. 8, pp. 159–236). Princeton, NJ: Princeton Universtiy Press.

Jung, C. G. (1952). Synchronicity: An acausal connecting principle. In *Collected works* (Vol. 8, pp. 417–531). Princeton, NJ: Princeton Universtiy Press.

Jung, C. G. (1954). The philosophical tree. In *Collected works* (Vol. 13, pp. 251–351). Princeton, NJ: Princeton University Press.

Jung, C. G. (2009). *The red book: Liber novus* (M. Kyburz & J. Peck, Trans., S. Shamdasani Ed.). New York & London: W. W. Norton & Company.

Kohut, H. (1977). *The restoration of the self*. New York: International Universities Press.

Laing, R. D. (1967). *The politics of experience*. New York: Pantheon Books.

Laszlo, E. (1996). *The systems view of the world*. Cresskill, NJ: Hampton Press.

Loewald, H. W. (1980). *Papers on psychoanalysis*. New Haven, CT: Yale University Press.

Maturana, J. M., & Varela, F. J. (1980). *Autopoiesis and cognition: The realization of the living*. Dordrecht: D. Reidel Publishing Company.

Perry, J. W. (2005). *The far side of madness*. Putnam, CT: Spring Publications.

Phillips, R. E., & Stein, C. H. (2007). God's will, god's punishment, or god's limitations: Religious coping strategies reported by young adults living with serious mental illness. *Journal of Clinical Psychology*, *63*, 529–540.

Rank, O. (1936). *Truth and reality: A life history of the human will*. New York: Alfred A. Knopf.

Read, J., van Os, J., Morrison, A., & Ross, C. (2005). Childhood trauma, psychosis and schizophrenia: A literature review with theoretical and clinical implications. *Acta Psychiatrica Scandinavica*, *112*, 330–350.

Shamdasani, S. (2008). 'The boundless expanse': Jung's reflections on life and death. *Quadrant: Journal of the C.G. Jung Foundation for Analytical Psychology*, *38*, 9–32.

Stern, D. B. (1997). *Unformulated experience: From dissociation to imagination in psychoanalysis*. Hillsdale, NJ: Analytic Press.

Sullivan, H. S. (1950). The illusion of personal individuality. In *The fusion of psychiatry and social science*. New York: W. W. Norton & Company.

Varela, F. J., Thompson, E., & Rosch, E. (1991). *The embodied mind: Cognitive science and human experience*. Cambridge, MA: MIT Press.

von Bertalanffy, L. (1968). *General systems theory*. New York: George Braziller.

Washburn, M. (1995). *The ego and the dynamic ground*. Albany, NY: SUNY Press.

Winnicott, D. W. (1971). *Playing and reality*. New York: Basic Books.

Witherington, D. C. (2011). Taking emergence seriously: The centrality of circular causality for dynamic systems approaches to development. *Human Development*, *54*, 66–92.

Chapter 2

Encounters with Sioux medicine men

Françoise Davoine

ABSTRACT: The author focuses on a series of encounters she and her husband had with Sioux medicine men during several summers on the Rosebud Reservation in South Dakota. In the company of these healers, the author and her husband shared clinical experiences on trauma and madness. From these encounters, the author learned Sioux teachings important for the conceptualization of madness, and of possible resonances these teachings had with psychoanalysis. In the same way that potters around the world use similar techniques to raise a pot around a central void – though the symbols carved or painted on the surface may vary – cross-cultural parallels can be drawn in our approaches to psychotherapy.

KEYWORDS: Lacan, psychoanalysis, Sioux, Renaissance literature, trauma

In his Tarner Lectures, which were given in 1956 at Trinity College, Cambridge, Nobel Prize winning quantum physicist Erwin Schrödinger launched an appeal to psychologists which I find useful in seeking to articulate an emancipatory perspective on madness. It occurs in a chapter titled "The Principle of Objectivation." Schrödinger writes:

> The material world has only been constructed at the price of taking the self, that is, mind, out of it, removing it; mind is not part of it; obviously, therefore, it can neither act on it nor be acted on by any of its parts.
>
> (Schrödinger, 1967, p. 128)

The stated intent of this great scientist is to free us from a worldview that is "colorless, cold, mute" (ibid). He writes that the world of science "has become so horribly objective as to leave no room for the mind and its immediate sensations" (p. 129). Schrödinger is explicit when he states:

> This sounds a paradox, but the wisest of all times and peoples have testified to confirm it. Men and women for whom this world was lit in an unusually bright light of awareness, and who by life and word have, more than others,

formed and transformed that work of art which we call humanity, testify by speech and writing or even by their very lives that more than others have they been torn by the pangs of inner discord. Let this be a consolation to him who also suffers from it. Without it nothing enduring has ever been begotten.

(p. 108)

Schrödinger's advice for contemporary psychotherapists is to effect a careful "blood transfusion" from those non-Western healing practices which have not separated mind from matter by way of "the initial gambit" reflected in excluding the psyche from the brain.

Starting in 1980, my husband, Jean Max Gaulillière, and I were to find ourselves following Schrödinger's suggestion. Over the course of several summers visiting the Rosebud Reservation located in South Dakota, we shared clinical experiences on trauma and madness with Sioux medicine men. This opportunity arose in context of a talk we gave at Austen Riggs Center in Stockbridge, Massachusetts. At that time, the psychoanalytic institute to which we belonged – the École Freudienne, founded by Jacques Lacan in Paris – endorsed what we considered to be a dated understanding of psychosis. The Lacanian orthodoxy contended that patients undergoing psychosis were unable to develop a transference. Objecting to this perspective, we were excited when an opportunity presented itself to visit Austen Riggs, where the psychoanalysis of psychosis was practiced in a different intellectual key.

We had been invited to Riggs to speak both on Lacan and on our weekly seminar entitled "Madness and the Social Link," which we offered at the École des Hautes Études en Sciences Sociales. In that seminar, it was our practice to present the ideas of an author dealing with madness in a transitional space between the more "objective" social sciences and the "psychotic transference" in which, as Schrödinger puts it, "the object is affected by our observation" (p. 135) – and hence the so-called neutral analyst by the patient.

An audience member, Jerry Mohatt, informed us of parallels he perceived between Lacan and the teachings of the Lakota people. Jerry was visiting from South Dakota with his wife Robby and their two kids. They lived on a ranch on the Rosebud Reservation and were part of the community. Jerry spoke the Lakota language and had participated in the creation of the Sinte Gleska college devoted to the teaching of Lakota culture. After hearing our talks among the staff at Riggs, he invited us to meet some Sioux medicine men: "for their speech is not so far from what your Lacan says." What did he mean? In order to answer that question, at the end of our stay at Riggs, we flew to Pierre, South Dakota, where Jerry was by then already waiting for us. We did not know what to expect, nor did we know anything about the Sioux people except through Hollywood Western movies.

Over the course of a number of summers, we participated in ceremonies and spoke with medicine men, especially Jerry's friend Joe Eagle Elk whose story is told in a book they wrote together (Mohatt & Eagle Elk, 2000). After several years, Jerry was appointed to the University of Alaska Fairbanks, where he invited us all to a conference. Meanwhile, Stanley Red Bird, an elder on the reservation, had formulated the wish to visit our country. So they came in 1985, to talk at our Institute in Paris and in the Maison de la Culture in Reims where we spent a week together, sharing our clinical experiences with the people of the town.

Stanley Red Bird told us: "What you are looking for here, you have it at home, perhaps lost along the way." We came to feel this was true. What did we learn that spoke to us at the crossroad between our cultures? In his "Remarks on Frazer's *The Golden Bough*," Wittgenstein (1933) writes: "in all these practices one, of course, sees something that is similar to the association of ideas and related to it. One could speak of an association of practices" (p. 145).

In the present context, I will develop several associations which became apparent between our practices and those of the Sioux people. I will tell stories that left a lasting impression, and which shaped my approach to working with patients.

Give away

The day after our arrival at Jerry's ranch on the reservation, he took us all some hundred miles away by the Missouri River to attend a Give Away. When we arrived, there were no pale faces except Jerry, Robby, their two boys, our own boys of the same age, and us. Dances had started to the rhythm of the drum, and songs were sung. At the center of the circle which had formed, an old woman was seated with younger men and women at her side. Before them was a heap of objects: some more obviously practical (saucepans, for example) and some more refined (such as patchwork blankets decorated with stars). After a while, the dancing stopped and we were invited to the tipi of a chief with a long feathered bonnet. He did not look at us until our kids dropped something and made a big noise, causing him to burst out in laughter. The convention of politeness was not to stare at us. This was intended to make us feel at ease. We were given food and the chief told us he had a French name, like many of his friends – Bordeaux Roubidou Beauvais. Then the dances started again. When they eventually reached their conclusion, all of the goods piled up in the middle were given away. I received a comb and my husband a pillow. Dollars were distributed to the dancers who were coming from far away.

Jerry explained to us that the people standing in the circle had lost a whole family in a car accident two years ago. They had accumulated sufficiently to Give Away their goods and depended now on their community to regain desire, strength, and regeneration. Jerry had correctly inferred a connection between this ceremony and the work of Lacan. While these were not Jerry's exact words, I understood that he saw a link with Lacan's theory on desire proceeding from a loss. In his seminar on "The Ethics of Psychoanalysis," Lacan (1959–60/1987) in fact cites the description of such a ritual named Potlatch on the West Coast offered by French anthropologist Marcel Mauss (1923/2016). In such ceremonies, one has to lose power in order to regain power.

In his seminar, Lacan draws a parallel with the munificent spending by noble families in the Middle Ages in order to receive, in turn, an increase of influence on others. I consider that in offering this example, Lacan misunderstood the notion of "power" adopted by the medicine men. For them, there is no counterpart, no countergift: "You, white people," Stanley Redbird used to say, "you are focused on accumulation. You do not understand the Give Away." That day, I perceived that what was at stake was the power of powerlessness as a condition for the regeneration of social links – not only with the community, but with the spirits of a land – threatened by a civilization that puts man at the top of the scale of beings and destroys the rest.

During critical sessions when our patients force us to experience powerlessness by making us fail, there is a chance for a new link to be created by acknowledging our blunders and monitoring our dreams. Only when we abandon our pretense to succeed with the patient's cure, only when we Give Away our professional qualities, can we reach the knowledge our patients paid so much to learn. Only then can we stand at the side of the patients and share the resources which help them in the crazy situations, when the laws of humanity have collapsed on the site of catastrophes and abuses which tore people from all trust in others. Medicine men call those helpers spirits. We call them voices or visions. They stem from an entrenched unconscious which speaks through things, animals, or trees, where human speech does not hold.

All my relatives

All my relatives, *Metakuye oyas'in*, is the formula you say when you are in a ceremony after the medicine man has communicated through his helpers, when everybody has to say something at his turn in the circle and you do not know what to say or you are too shy to speak. At first, I thought that "relatives" referred specifically to the parental lineage, but it means all things to which I am related. This includes animals, plants, and the wider landscape. The scale of being for the Sioux is opposite of the Western one, where man is at the top of the pyramid. The order is the other way round. On the top are the rocks who do not need the plants to live, then the plants who do not need the animals (except the bees), then the animals who do not need humans. We humans are at the bottom.

This hierarchy is paramount for patients who do not trust humans any more after having been betrayed. One of the definitions of trauma is the betrayal by one's own people – by one's own command during the war, by people at the rear, by your parents, or by your friends and neighbors. We usually overlook the help that little things like plants or animals offer to our patients, when words can no longer be trusted.

A man was in a delusion. He told me that he had been raised in Mexico. At 6 years old, his parents decided to return to France. They sent him by himself on an Air France plane with his dog. Waiting for him at the airport in Paris was his grandfather, whom he had never met. When they landed, the dog was dead, choked in the luggage hold. The grandfather showed no reaction to the boy's loss. Following this incident, the boy refused to learn French and had difficulties in school. I told the man who had once been the boy that we could consider that the dog had given away his life so that he may survive in France. Why did I say that? I did not know. At the same time, I took from my shelf a framed photograph of a Saint Bernard dog and I told the man that this dog had saved my mother's life in the mountains, a year before my birth, and had died of a heart attack immediately after. I owed my life to the dog's sacrifice.

We often despise, as symptomatic, the little things to which our patients are related for their survival when humans have treated them like nothing. The art historian Aby Warburg became mad during World War I. He was confined in Switzerland in the clinic of Sigmund Freud's disciple Ludwig Binswanger (1921). There he was raving mad, to the point that it was thought his mind was lost forever. He used to speak to his dear soap, his dear carpet, and to the moths which he considered the souls of the dead. Psychosis, in his case, sensed the danger of rising anti-Semitism, which he had already witnessed as a child in the aftermath of the previous Franco-Prussian War of 1870, where Jews started to be considered like *untermensch*. Prior to his recovery, he cried out in the clinic, in 1922, that all the Jews would be exterminated. The medicine man would say that the spirits had spoken.

The animistic world

"Speak to the raven," say Native people in Alaska. That's what I did, after my grandmother's death, when a crow came at my window. My grandmother hadn't said she would go to paradise or purgatory, but to the land of her relatives, which included not only her ancestors but the spirits of her land – animals, herbs, and places which remained vivid for her years after she had to leave them.

I remember a meeting that Jerry Mohatt organized on Manitoulin Island, Ontario, in 1988, between Sioux and Ojibwe elders, a number of psychoanalysts, and several anthropologists. I told the story of a delusional young girl who brought pansies to her mother's grave in order to share her thoughts, for in French *pensées* mean thoughts. After the coffee break, a lady called Sara Smith came to me. She said: "The proof that the spirits speak through her mouth is that flower, which is a real thought." At that time I was not familiar with what Bion (1992, p. 309) calls "thoughts without a thinker" which "are things, as things are thoughts", or with what Aby Warburg calls "surviving images" (see Didi-Huberman, 2016) – speaking beyond the law of language when the warrants of human speech have been destroyed.

Sara Smith introduced herself as an Iroquois potter coming from the neighbor territory of the Six Nations. She told me: "After terrible wars between our tribes, we buried our weapons under a tree and created a Confederation. I am Mohawk and I can tell you that the roots of that tree spread to the four directions. You came along the root spreading to the East, and I thank you for that." I was stunned to become suddenly an Eastern pilgrim.

When clinicians come for supervision, I always ask them where their patients come from. Often the answer I receive is vague. They come from Africa, or from somewhere in the countryside which is virtually as unknown to the therapist as Africa. I then advise them to bring a map and look for geographic details with their patients and with the parents of children who come to therapy. I ask for the names, not only of the villages, but of the fields, of the woods, of the rocks, of the mountains which speak to their ancestors. When my patients are speechless, I tell them stories or quote songs of long ago. This is also true in the United States, where the lands from which people fled in exile after major catastrophes in Europe or elsewhere bear witness of slaughters and abuses that return in the speech of delusional descendants.

The stories I tell, the songs I mention – and even sing – connect to a common lore of very long ago. We could say that the spirits of the land speak through the music. During World War II, a musicologist, Paul Davenson, was taken prisoner. He collected old French songs and managed to pass them underground, to keep the French soul alive while the Nazi totalitarian power threatened to overwhelm it. They were published, during the war, in Switzerland (Davenson, 1941–43). By telling my stories and my songs, I disclose something – something we were not allowed to do in orthodox psychoanalysis.

Sioux ceremonies emphasize the importance of the drum and the song. In psychoanalysis, we cannot work if we do not establish a rhythm in the deadly stoppage of time, brought by our patients, from areas of death, where they have been attacked by a ruthless agency whose aim is to destroy all their links. When my patients cannot speak, stories and songs, also dreams, come to my mind, as if they were whispered to my ears, and I have to disclose them.

Disclosure

At the beginning of a ceremony, the medicine man Joe Eagle Elk used to talk of the vision that put him on the path of becoming a medicine man. Rarely do analysts quote such an episode which threw them on the path of psychoanalysis. Still, when we deal with psychosis or trauma, we are often stunned by interferences, triggered by patients' delusions, with discarded parts of our own story. Why not disclose that meeting which does not belong to us, but comes from beyond us? My experience is that this disclosure is the only means to move time into motion when it has been put out of joint in some area of catastrophe. It took me a long time to connect with a vision of my childhood which pushed me on the path of psychoanalysis. An important ritual among the Sioux is called the Vision Quest.

When I was around 8 years old, every Monday morning I told my best friend, while bicycling on the way to school, that I had spent the weekend with a young man in a blue uniform. I knew it was not true, but at the same time, that there was a truth in it. In later life, I never spoke of this to my Lacanian psychoanalyst for fear that he would think I was crazy. In my 60s, I asked my aged father: what was I doing during my first two years in our home situated in the Alps in a war zone, where the underground used to meet? He answered right away: "You attended the meetings quietly. There were two men who wore the blue uniform of a collaborationist organization – they were gathering intelligence for the Resistance. One of them loved you. He always took you on his lap. He must have had a child of your age. One day, he was caught. I saw him between two German soldiers, awfully tortured. He looked at me. I saw his gaze. Every day I see his blue eyes. His name was Vitek and he was Jewish. They shot him soon after."

Before I knew the identity of this man who died without a grave, he had helped me to identify the ghosts haunting a delusional patient in the psychiatric hospital where I worked as a psychoanalyst. Her father had been the only survivor of the massacre of his companions during a battle. My father also survived a massacre. At that time, I did not dare to disclose anything. One day, she came saying that the extraterrestrials had visited her and asked her to come back to them. I knew that she was on the verge of committing suicide, and I guessed that the extraterrestrials were her father's companions who had been left rotting on the ground. So to speak, my companion in the blue uniform suggested my answer. Not by the way of something objective. I knew that if I had said, no wonder, the extraterrestrials are the souls of the slaughtered boys, she would have answered, I know, but so what? I said: "Time does not flow for them as it does for us. A week may mean many years." She answered: "Oh! Einstein's relativity!" And her delusions stopped. What worked, of course, was not a scientific knowledge, but the interference between two entrenched historical truths – one on her side and the other on mine.

Long after, I had a strange experience at the Veterans' hospital in Miami where I was giving a talk at a conference on "the Veterans' transmission to their descendants." This was after my father had disclosed the name of my childhood lover. There, I told that story for the first time. At the coffee break, a young woman introduced herself, Deborah. Her parents were friends with Vitek's wife who had emigrated to the United States after the war, and I learned from her that Vitek's wife had a boy of my age. I was stunned, out of Time, and had to return to the speakers' table. I didn't have time to ask her full name or get her contact details. At the end of the conference, I looked for her without success. Like a messenger of the gods in the ancient Greek time who appears to Odysseus and then disappears, I still look for her, thinking of this man my age who perhaps did not know that his father was in the resistance under the cover of his blue uniform. Never say: "no wonder."

Now I can tell, the ghosts of my history have been my helpers. Bion had the same experience after he was past 70, exiling himself in Los Angeles. Only then did he dare to acknowledge that his helpers, when he worked with psychotic patients, were the spirits of his dead comrades, when, at 20 years old, he was the captain of a tank unit during World War I. He meets one of them in the end of the second part of *A Memoir of the Future*, entitled "The Past Presented" (Bion, 1991, p. 423). When the ghost asks him if he is happy to see him again, the psychoanalyst answers: "Indeed, but I was afraid to meet you."

We are indeed afraid to meet – the land of the marvel

In the Middle Ages, the mad person could talk to fairies, animals, plants, and rocks, and fight monsters, in an arrested time, about which they tried to bear witness through voices and visions of fake discourses in the normal social link. Today, Joan of Arc – who received her voices and visions while she was a shepherdess near a tree called the Fairy Tree – would be treated with drugs and shocks.

Others took refuge in literature, without which we would never know they existed. *Don Quixote* appeared to Cervantes (1605) when he was put in jail in Sevilla at age 45. Cervantes had fought at war for five years in his youth and been enslaved for five more in Alger. The crazy knight helped him to confront his own ghost that he had left in Algeria, embodied in the novel by a captive who comes back after his escape from slavery.

Don Quixote makes us laugh – a feature also of the Sioux ceremonies. When I asked for a ceremony on the behalf of my mother who was diagnosed with cancer, I had to cook a lot of food for the participants. The medicine man had ordered a beef tongue, as I was a foreigner, but the rest was traditional fare: fried bread and *wajapi*, a jam of chalk cherries. When the lights were switched on again – for they were out during the ritual – I went around with my pans, distributing the food, while jokes burst out. As these jokes were told in Lakota, I was given the translation. Some were dirty jokes which reminded me of François Rabelais, who, during the 16th century, was also a physician – a medicine man. He writes: "Better it is to write about laughter than about sorrow, for laughter is man's own" (Rabelais, 1552, Ch. LV, author's translation).

Laughter warms up the frozen words which have been cut out and kept intact in the spirit world. In the fourth book of Rabelais's story, the giant Pantagruel and his friends, the fool Panurge and the warrior monk, are at sea, when they hear voices. The captain informs them that on that spot, a fierce battle was fought the previous winter on the icy waters. Suddenly, hailstones of different colors fall on the deck. The seafarers warm them in their hands, thus freeing frozen speeches: the words of cutthroats, the cries of children and women, the neighing of horses and the din of weapons. All may at last be acknowledged. Subsequent to this, they do not linger in the gloom but share a joyful banquet and laugh.

When I am asked "what did you learn from the Sioux medicine man?" I can only say: "I learned to laugh," which was a relief – especially when psychoanalysis seems so deadly serious. Of course, we laughed at Lacan's puns, but we feared to criticize him. In the Middle Ages, jesters could be hanged when they made fun of the authorities' pretense.

I remember a dialogue with Stanley Red Bird when he started to attack me: "You white people, you gave us promises and instead fed us with lies." I retorted: "Look Stanley, I am not the white people." He did not let me finish and burst out into laughter: "I just wished to test your fake culpability!"

It might be suggested that the psychoanalytic psychotherapy of madness and trauma is the form taken in our culture to create a place for the praise of folly when it is threatened by objectification. Thanks to the encounter with an analyst, who Dori Laub characterizes as "a witness for events without a witness" (Laub & Felmann, 1992, p. 75), and with which we might draw a Homeric parallel in the notion of a *therapon*, the second in combat, and the ritual double in charge of funeral duties (see Nagy, 1979, pp. 292–293) – folly may claim "unclaimed experiences" (Caruth, 1996) denied by ruthless agencies, and take care of those who have disappeared. By telling untold stories and singing unsung songs, a freedom of speech is opened for voices and visions, which give birth to a "Political self" (Tweedy, 2017) on the site of destruction. Instead of being reduced to the treatment of individual symptoms, we may claim the legacy expressed by Socrates to Phaedrus when he contests that delusion is a pathological symptom:

> On the contrary, among our good things, one of the best comes through a delusion which is a divine gift . . . When old intergenerational wraths express themselves through an individual, he may free not only himself but all of his relatives, by participating in healing ceremonies which will transform madness, *mania* into *mantikè*, the art of divination, by adding a "t" coming from the word *istôria*.
>
> (Plat. Phaed. § 244, author's translation)

References

Binswanger, L. (1921). *Freud's correspondence*, 8 Nov. 1921. Paris: Calmann Levy, 1995.

Bion, W. (1991). *A memoir of the future*. London: Karnac Books.

Bion, W. (1992). *Cogitations*. London: Karnac Books.

Caruth, C. (1996). *Unclaimed experience*. Baltimore & London: Johns Hopkins University Press.

Cervantes (1605). *Don Quixote* (J. Rutherford, Trans.). New York: Penguin, 2005.

Davenson, P. (1941–43). *Introduction à la chanson française*. Neuchâtel, Switzerland: Editions de la Baconnière.

Didi-Huberman, G. (2016). *The surviving image: Phantoms of time and time of phantoms: Aby Warburg's history of art*. University Park, PA: Penn State University Press.

Lacan, J. (1959–1960/1987). *The ethics of psychoanalysis*. New York: W. W. Norton & Company.

Laub, D., & Felmann, S. (1992). *Testimony*. London: Routledge.

Mauss, M. (1923/2016). *Essay on the gift* (J. Guyer, Trans.). Chicago, IL: University of Chicago Press.

Mohatt, G., & Eagle Elk, J. (2000). *The price of a gift, a Lakota Healer's story*. Lincoln: University of Nebraska Press.

Nagy, G. (1979). *The best of the Acheans*. Baltimore & London: John Hopkins University Press.

Rabelais, F. (1552). *Quart livre*.

Schrödinger, E. (1967). *Mind and matter*. Cambridge: Cambridge University Press.

Tweedy, R. (2017). *The political self*. London: Karnac Books.

Wittgenstein, L. (1933/1997). Remarks on Frazer's golden bough. In J. C. Klagge & A. Nordmann (Eds.), *Philosophical occasions* (pp. 118–155). Indianapolis: Hackett Publishing Company.

Chapter 3

Transpersonal enactments and the teleology of paranoia

Robin S. Brown and Marie Brown

ABSTRACT: This chapter questions definitions of mental health that implicitly assume the separation of self and world to be normative. We consider the importance of C.G. Jung's synchronicity principle as a means to thinking less reductively about madness. This possibility emerges with recent developments in the field of psychoanalysis as reflected most centrally in the notion of enactment. We offer a radical interpretation of enactment in light of Jung's synchronicity principle. This line of thinking posits a re-enchanted conception of the world with deepseated implications for the understanding of madness. In support of this approach, we offer an extended example of a case of *folie à famille*. This case illustrates how a shared paranoia within a family served the purpose of forging connections to a disavowed Sámi heritage. We use this example to demonstrate how paranoia or "madness" can be understood to have a teleological function. Madness is here described as a vehicle for personal, familial, and collective healing.

KEYWORDS: enactment, intergenerational trauma, paranoia, synchronicity, teleology, transpersonal

Our understanding of madness is dependent upon our assumptions about reality. Since the Enlightenment, these assumptions have come to be shaped most obviously by the claims of empirical science. The scientific method offers a compelling basis from which to establish *facts* about the reality apparently disclosed to us by the senses. With the accumulation of these facts and their functional value in effecting material change, the scientific gestalt holds powerful sway over the popular imagination. Since its inception, modern science has offered itself as a basis for emancipation from religious dogma – one which enables disputes to be settled without recourse to unreasoned faith and the authority of a religious elite. Yet, this narrative has tended to occlude recognition of the significant respects in which the scientific method inevitably rests upon principles than cannot themselves be confirmed via the scientific method. With the extent to which our understanding of reality has come to be informed by the claims upon which the scientific method rests, it is critical that these claims be carefully appraised lest their habitual nature come to mask expressions of violence toward those modes of experience labeled mad.

In the present context, we will focus on the theme of *isolation*. Progressive approaches to psychosis have often emphasized the necessity of situating madness within social context. R.D. Laing's (1959) pithy formulation that madness reflects a sane response to an insane situation typifies this important line of thinking. Isolating mad individuals as the object of psychiatric inquiry entails a fundamental distortion of the phenomenon in question. This tendency is nowhere more evident than when mental or emotional suffering and/or difference is interpreted as a consequence of biology. When we insist upon understanding individuals within their wider social context, new possibilities for meaning emerge. Madness is registered more comprehensible. This can have enormous value in alleviating distress and facilitating understanding. Nevertheless, such an approach may yet be accused of a more subtle kind of reductivism. Madness in this scheme of thinking is liable to be seen as a necessary lean-to when an individual's context denies them the opportunity to experience and communicate "normally." While this is certainly a more empathic frame of reference than the one offered by the biomedical model, it still tends to perpetuate a sense that madness reflects a distortion of reality, even if the latent content of these experiences has meaning.

Addressing this shortcoming requires that we go further in examining the role of isolation in our thinking. It is endemic to good scientific practice that the object of study be isolated. The distinction between the hard and soft sciences largely depends upon the extent to which isolating variables is deemed practicable. In challenging the biomedical desire to treat individuals in isolation, an approach that stresses understanding the individual's immediate social context reflects a significant step forward. Yet in understanding madness in these terms, an isolation is still apparent between the observer and the wider context now observed. For example, in shifting focus from the individual to the family system much is no doubt gained; yet, it might be objected that such an approach still isolates the family.

Broadening our field of observation will only take us so far if we fail to include the concept of the observer. The clinical gaze mediates our standards of sanity. In a therapeutic situation, the role of the observer is played by the clinician. Within psychoanalytic theory, the domain of countertransference has been circumscribed in an effort to address this. Classically, countertransference is understood to be a distortion wherein the clinician's subjectivity potentially occludes a more correct view of the patient. Thus, addressing the clinician's role in supporting the patient's condition means monitoring oneself via self-observation. A split is thus upheld between the clinician's participation and a capacity to withhold from intruding. The undertaking to address the clinician's role is therefore merely to reinforce the need that they remain distinct from the patient. The problem with this approach becomes apparent when we realize that the clinical definition of madness hinges upon affirming just this distinction – the hallmark of madness is considered to be the incapacity to separate oneself from the other. A paranoid disposition is betrayed whenever one's capacity to see things as they are appears jeopardized by the imposition of one's subjectivity.

Disenchantment

Post-Enlightenment science has been founded in a belief that it is possible to withdraw one's projections via the experimental method. In the 20th century, these assumptions were challenged by developments in the field of quantum physics. At the quantum level, the act of observation is understood to unavoidably effect the results obtained. For some, this phenomenon has seemed to offer support in questioning the assumptions of science more broadly. We see this reflected in the words of Werner Heisenberg:

> The positivists have a simple solution: the world must be divided into that which we can say clearly and the rest, which we had better pass over in silence. But can anyone conceive of a more pointless philosophy, seeing that what we can say clearly amounts to next to nothing? If we omitted all that is unclear we would probably be left with completely uninteresting and trivial tautologies.
>
> (1971, p. 208)

Despite the challenges posed by quantum physics, "good" scientific practice has continued to pride itself on isolating the observer from the observed. For this reason, the scientific standards of the biomedical model naturally require that a paranoid outlook be considered abnormal, and the capacity to separate oneself from the other comes to be considered the barometer of mental health. This definition of madness is required so as to maintain the sanity of Western science's reified conception of truth – this being reflected in the sense of an unchanging objective reality founded on a steadily accumulating dossier of facts.

Max Weber (1963) adopted the term disenchantment (*Entzauberung*) from Friederich Schiller to reflect the fashion in which scientific belief has resulted in a secularized society. With an emerging faith that science will ultimately be able to answer all the big questions along objective and rational lines, religious or folk beliefs are eroded. Accompanying this tendency is a loss of communal belonging, an emphasis on private experience, and the rise of widespread alienation. The condition of disenchantment is perhaps liable to be understood as an inevitable side effect of scientific progress, in which light it is readily assumed that disenchantment reflects a more true (because more objective) mode of consciousness. What this fails to register is that scientific positivism postulates disenchantment as normative from the outset. This is quite clear in the foundational assumption that the object can be observed in isolation from the subject. In other words, disenchantment is not an innocent byproduct of scientific progress so much as an ideological demand on consciousness.

Disenchantment is of central importance with regard to the evaluation of madness as a spiritual phenomenon – a matter which is insufficiently emphasized in the literature. Where spirituality is positively linked with outcomes in respect to psychosis, spirituality tends to be understood as a "protective factor." Spiritual concerns are in effect treated as beliefs that can aid recovery. What this potentially neglects is the *experiential* basis upon which these beliefs often rest. Within the discipline of transpersonal psychology this tendency is often challenged, and madness is linked more directly to the idea of spiritual awakening. One of the most significant contributions in this direction has been offered by Stanislav Grof, whose work with psychedelic-assisted psychotherapy and Holotropic Breathwork has done much to connect breaking down with breaking through. Even Grof, however, has drawn a distinction between "medical psychosis" and what he terms "spiritual emergency":

> Many mental disorders are directly related to brain dysfunctions or diseases of other organs and systems of the body. A good medical and psychiatric examination is, therefore, a necessary prerequisite for any alternative therapeutic considerations. When these examinations do not detect any medical cause, the decision will depend on the nature of the client's experiences, attitude toward the process, the experiential style, and ability to relate and cooperate. Even individuals who would otherwise meet the criteria of having a spiritual emergency cannot be treated by or benefit from the new strategies if they are unable to see their problems as related to an inner process, or are unwilling to undergo the pain of confronting the underlying experiences.
>
> (Grof & Grof, 2017, p. 31)

We believe that this distinction is problematic. Such an approach suffers from arbitrarily separating "symptomatic delusion" from authentic spirituality. This distinction is ultimately founded in an individual's success in being able to communicate their experience and hence remains tied to a "reality-based" approach that only tolerates the other's condition without pathologizing in so far as madness remains relatable. This tendency is reflective of a conception of fundamental reality which implicitly reinforces the Cartesian separation of person and world, this being reflected in an emphasis on interiority and the capacity to appropriately experience oneself in these terms. In response to this tendency, Jorge Ferrer has initiated a revisioning of transpersonal studies which has been centrally concerned with critiquing what he terms *subtle Cartesianism*. The participatory framework Ferrer (2002) offers seeks to emphasize the interdependence of subject and object:

> aspects belonging to the structures of subjectivity can reach out and become, in a way, objects for consciousness in the external world. Of course, the

defense mechanism of projection comes rapidly to mind in this regard. However, psychodynamic accounts of projection are not helpful in explaining the idea to be grasped here, because they depict this external objectification of the subjective as an intrapsychic phenomenon: The projection of our repressed feelings or unconscious personality traits upon people or events does not really transform them; what changes is only our experience of them. By contrast, in transpersonal and spiritual development . . . new worlds of corresponding objects and meanings *actually* emerge as consciousness evolves and identifies itself with new structures of subjectivity. This idea receives support from many contemplative traditions such as Vajrayana Buddhism or Kabbalah, which maintain that inner spiritual practices are not merely aimed at changing the self, but at the actual transformation of the world.

(p. 31, italics in original)

Ferrer asserts that the emphasis transpersonal psychology has tended to place on transformative *experiences* tends to semantically privilege interiority, and that we might be better served in speaking of transformative *events*. The participatory nature of spirituality is thus emphasized, and transpersonal phenomena can be understood not only as inner experiences but also in terms of our relationships to others, the environment, and the wider cosmos.

Enactment and madness

The theme of participation has also come to assume a central role in the development of North American psychoanalysis. Of fundamental importance in this respect is the idea of *enactment* and its evolving exposition within the psychoanalytic literature. This concept can be understood in relationship to the notion of *acting out*. In the earlier history of psychoanalysis, acting out is a term adopted to signify the way in which an individual repetitiously performs unresolved aspects of past experience as a consequence of the failure to transform this experience into words and hence be able to properly reflect upon it. This tendency was often understood as a form of resistance to treatment; rather than talking about their transference fantasies, patients acted upon them.

With the recognition of countertransference, it also became possible to identify how analysts are themselves not immune to acting out. The concept of enactment has emerged over the last thirty years to describe the fashion in which one party's acting out (emphasis typically on the patient) elicits a complementary acting out in the other (emphasis typically on the analyst). Under such circumstances, patient and analyst join to play out a shared drama that is reflective of their past experiences, and of which both remain largely unconscious.

Enactment was initially understood to reflect episodic disruptions to the treatment wherein patient and analyst collude to create a therapeutic impasse out of their mutual resistances. This episodic conception of enactment has been increasingly challenged, however, with a recognition that patient and analyst alike are *constantly* influencing each other in ways that are unconscious. It has therefore been suggested that rather than approaching enactment in episodic terms, we might more correctly think of enactment as a constant factor in therapeutic work. In this light, it seems sensible to suppose that enactment is by no means inherently destructive. Enactment becomes problematic where the treatment falls into an impasse such that the parties must somehow become aware of the unconscious dynamics that have gotten them stuck. Many relational analysts have increasingly come to believe that there is actually something healing about the enactive process itself, and that while some forms of enactment are destructive, others can be creative (Aron & Atlas, 2015). Unconsciously recapitulating past experiences in the treatment can be healing when the participants are able to bring about a different sort of outcome.

How does the idea of enactment shape our understanding of madness? The initial significance lies in the extent to which this notion underscores the reciprocal embedded nature of unconscious processes. Attributions of madness tend to reflect a perception that a particular individual is less in touch with reality. The idea of enactment is helpful in promoting a recognition of the role that might be played by the "sane" party (or parties) in keeping the "insane" crazy (and vice-versa). In a clinical context, it might be supposed that reaching the mad person wouldn't mean fixing their wrong attitude, but rather attempting to become aware of our own participation in sustaining the other's apparently unreachable condition; this being reflected in the propensity to impose order on experience by perceiving the other person as merely crazy.

Perhaps the mad person's apparent inability or unwillingness to separate self from other can be considered an invitation to participate. In conformity with many Indigenous healing practices, the idea that enactment can be a creative process may lead us to better understand why madness is not to be challenged but rather joined with. In light of enactment, the commonplace fear of "colluding" with the patient is thrown into an altogether different light. In opposing the other person's madness as madness, we more often than not merely enact something of the dynamic that brought this person to the place where they currently stand. In imposing our own notions of reason or reality, we merely reinforce the other person's status as senseless. In realizing that collusion is inevitable, clinicians might start to ask how to collude more creatively. This entails recognizing madness not only as a potentially transformative process for the person identified as being mad, but also for those who would seek to engage them.

The notion of enactment is thus helpful in elucidating the work of Harold Searles, who posited that all psychopathology is an effect of the patient's frustrated efforts to heal others. In seeking to explain why clincinans *must* be transformed by their patients, Slavin and Kriegman (1998) suggest that we might think of the transference as a probe that should ultimately result in the analyst's own subjectivity being more fully realized within the treatment. When the analyst shows a willingness to confront his or her own conflicts and change in light of interactions with the patient, the authors argue that this malleability and willingness to be affected provides the essential therapeutic experience. From their work with psychotic patients, Davoine and Gaudillière (2004) add a critical element to our understanding of this process. They argue that in order to make therapeutically meaningful contact with the patient, the essential element is provided by an uncanny coincidence in the generational histories of trauma associated with both patient and clinician. Only in thus discovering a break in the deterministic hold of reason does the possibility of effecting a genuine change emerge. We consider that further examining the role of coincidence is essential in seeking to realize a more adequate (i.e. less reductive) conception of enacted process.

Relevance of the synchronicity principle

How is the "unconscious communication" in enactment understood to be accomplished? For some analysts, it is considered adequate to interpret this phenomenon merely in terms of the innumerable subtle behavioral cues exchanged between patient and analyst. However, clinicians have often been struck by the sometimes uncanny nature of meaningful coincidences occurring in the context of treatment. The notion of "unconscious orchestration" and the potentially constructive nature of that orchestration invites psychoanalysis to engage more directly with themes that are liable to be associated with spirituality.

We might seek to understand the uncanny aspect of enactment in terms of Jung's notion of synchronicity. The synchronicity principle reflects an undertaking to account for the existence of moments of meaningful coincidence between the inner life of individuals and the external world. One of Jung's most often referenced examples of synchronicity is given as follows:

My example concerns a young woman patient who, in spite of efforts made on both sides, proved to be psychologically inaccessible. The difficulty lay in the fact that she always knew better about everything. Her excellent education had provided her with a weapon ideally suited to this purpose, namely a highly polished Cartesian rationalism with an impeccably "geometrical" idea of reality. After several fruitless attempts to sweeten her rationalism with a somewhat more human understanding, I had to confine myself to the hope that something unexpected and irrational would turn up, something that would burst the intellectual retort into which she had sealed herself. Well, I was sitting opposite her one day, with my back to the window, listening to her flow of rhetoric. She had an impressive dream the night before, in which someone had given her a golden scarab – a costly piece of jewelry. While she was still telling me this dream, I heard something behind me gently tapping on the window. I turned round and saw that it was a fairly large flying insect that was knocking against the window-pane from outside in the obvious effort to get into the dark room. This seemed to me very strange. I opened the window immediately and caught the insect in the air as it flew in. It was a scarabaeid beetle, or common rose-chafer (*Cetonia aurata*), whose gold-green color most nearly resembles that of a golden scarab. I handed the beetle to my patient with the words, "Here is your scarab." This experience punctured the desired hole in her rationalism and broke the ice of her intellectual resistance. The treatment could now be continued with satisfactory results.

(1952, para. 982)

While the notion of enactment focuses on meaningful coincidence between subjects in their unconscious relatedness, the emphasis in synchronicity lies with a broader correspondence between psyche and matter. In order to gain a more adequate picture of how enactment functions, it is helpful if we supplement this body of theory with Jung's more abstract ideas about synchronicity. Doing so better allows us to understand the uncanny elements of enacted process as reflected not only in the specificity of fit between patient and analyst, but also in terms of material events transpiring both inside and, more comprehensively, *outside* the treatment.

Jung's explicit theoretical elaboration of the synchronicity principle was relatively limited. He did little to examine this concept in relationship to the function of clinical work or the nature of interpersonal relatedness more broadly. His focus was on positing this idea in terms of the latest developments in physics – he believed that the notion of meaningful coincidence between a human subject (the observer) and the external environment (the observed) suggested a basic compatibility with quantum physics. Jung's work on synchronicity has also tended to foreground the more striking examples. This is understandable, given that his initial concern was for having this phenomenon simply be understood and accepted as posing a legitimate question for science. However, it has been suggested that this emphasis is perhaps misleading, and that synchronicity was intended to be understood as a governing principle that substantially shapes our daily experience (Progoff, 1973; von Franz, 1980).

A transpersonal notion of enactment draws attention to the possible function of synchronicity as a constant factor mediating our relatedness to the world. Correspondingly, Jung's notion of synchronicity helps us better recognize the enacted dimension of daily living. It is in this fashion that the idea of enactment can be understood in terms of disenchantment. The participatory vision of human relatedness that emerges out of this radically challenges the legitimacy of postulating the capacity to separate subject from object as the marker of mental health. Such an outlook might be employed so as to challenge the tendency to consider paranoia as expressive of a subjective overlay on an objective reality. In this fashion, we might seek to radically expand Slavin and Kriegman's (1998) notion of the transference as a probe by suggesting that a paranoid attitude can be understood not merely as an interpersonal instigation, but as a kind of metaphysical yearning.

Paranoia would then reflect an urgent attempt to realize a more enchanted mode of relationship to the environment such as to effectuate collective healing.

A case example

As a child, Anja grew up in a house at the edge of a winding river. The house was built on what had once been Native American land. Although, of course, all North American land can be considered Native American, the site upon which Anja's childhood home had been built was sufficiently noteworthy as to have been the location of an archeological dig conducted by the local university's anthropology department. The findings were featured in a book, long since out of print. Anja's neighbors owned a copy which they would sometimes take down off the shelf so that she could look at the images of broken pottery and bones, each photograph neatly labeled in ink. Playing in the yard, Anja and her brother would periodically find arrowheads pushing up through the earth. Anja's father would often stare dreamily out the back window, telling the family about the Native American ghosts he saw. Anja never saw a Native American ghost herself, but sometimes in bed, late at night, she thought that she could hear them.

Within contemporary psychoanalytic discourse, ghosts are often evoked metaphorically. Fraiberg, Adelson, and Shapiro (1975) discuss the ways in which past familial traumas, such as abuse and neglect, can "haunt" infant-caregiver bonds. They state, "While no one has issued an invitation, the ghosts take up residence and conduct the rehearsal of the family tragedy from a tattered script" (p. 388). In their introduction to *Ghosts in the Consulting Room: Echos of Trauma in Psycho-analysis*, editors Harris, Kalb, and Klebanoff (2016) describe ghosts as unmetabolized or unprocessed experiences that cause disturbances within communities, bodies, interpersonal relationships, and intrapsychic life. Psychoanalytically speaking, ghosts can be understood as unconscious influences arising from painful experiences which were never openly acknowledged, witnessed, or named.

When Anja was a child, her family believed that a local government agency called the Department of Land Acquisitions (DLA) had a personal vendetta against her father and that their home was under threat. This belief centered on the idea that the DLA was interested in gaining control over their property due to the proximity of the house to a waterway. Anja was told to never answer the door to strangers in fear that it might be a DLA agent. Her father posted huge "No Trespassing" signs all over the yard and spoke of conducting a "citizen's arrest" if anyone from the DLA stepped foot on the property. During that time, it seemed that helicopters flew relentlessly overhead – a sign, her father said, of the DLA's constant surveillance of the land. He painted the doors to the house a bright red to further underscore the warning: "Keep Out." Now an adult, Anja has vague memories from that time of strange men with flashlights walking around the yard at night, her father emerging from the darkness, shotgun in hand, full of boasts having thwarted yet another DLA agent's nefarious activity.

According to the *DSM-5* (American Psychiatric Association, 2013), "shared delusions" occur as a type of contagion. An individual's persecutory delusions are transferred to one or more susceptible individuals with whom they have a close emotional bond. When this occurs within an entire family, it is sometimes referred to by the term *folie à famille*. Such occurrences are often thought to serve the function of stabilizing family tensions and aggression by creating a common bond against an outside enemy (Wexler, 1992). To some degree, this was the case with Anja's family during childhood. However, as she grew older and began to socialize outside of the house more, she began to believe less and less in the DLA. Home was a largely dysfunctional and violent place, so Anja spent more and more time away, attempting to construct her own "family" with other social misfits. Although she never thought the notion of the DLA's hostility was entirely fabricated, she began to question the level of investment the DLA had in her family and land. After all, what made her family so special? What did they have against her father specifically? Why didn't they have the same investment in the other homes along the river?

As the years went on, tensions within her home continued to build. Her father succumbed to alcoholism and violent rage, while her mother lost herself in work outside the home. Her brother slowly became less of a presence in the household and, by the time Anja graduated high school, she was already profoundly addicted to heroin. All the while, her family lived awash in the relentless monologue of her father's fiery indignation toward the DLA.

Throughout Anja's life, her Sámi roots were something largely unspoken of except in occasional fragments and hearsay. She knew her father's family arrived in the country as galley cook staff that had jumped ship at the US shoreline. Her father did not know the names of his grandparents. When Anja asked questions about her ethnicity, there was always the vague response of "Scandinavian," which later became "Finnish." She remembers feeling there was something odd or embarrassing about inquiring further.

The Sámi are the Indigenous peoples of Sápmi, or what is now considered northern Europe, inclusive of Finland, Norway, Sweden, and Russia. Like the Indigenous peoples of North America, the Sámi have similarly been subject to systematic persecution, colonization, assimilation, and forced removal from their ancestral land. In the 14th and 15th centuries, Sámi people were prohibited from practicing their religion and were at risk of being burned at the stake for witchcraft if caught doing so. Beginning in the 19th century, many Sámi children were taken from their parents and placed in European boarding schools where they were forbidden to speak their mother tongue and denied access to their cultural traditions. Seen as inferior to their European counterparts, the Sámi were victims of eugenics practices, such as forced sterilization. Within this hostile climate, many Sámi people sought to assimilate into European culture by disavowing their ethnicity and cultural heritage and adopting that of their oppressors. As a group largely Caucasian in appearance, it was easy to "pass" as European, particularly when living outside of Scandinavia. It is from this historical context that Anja's paternal lineage arrived in the United States.

Davoine and Gaudillière (2004) extend the metaphor of ghosts and hauntings to the concept of madness, viewing madness (or "psychosis") as having a direct relationship to unspoken mass historical traumas, including war and genocide. Such traumas result in an atemporality, freezing an individual within catastrophic circumstances that cannot be remembered. They state, "The past is present, the dead return. It is a child's voice that is speaking . . . through the mouth of the adult he has become, in the name of an entire society threatened with disappearance" (p. xxvii). Davoine & Gaudillière's ideas about psychosis help make sense of Anja's family's madness. Emanating from her father, perhaps the "paranoid delusion" of the government stealing their land can be understood as a ghostly dispatch from the unremembered past of their Sámi ancestors, a past occurring in the present because it was never inscribed in time to begin with. Davoine & Gaudillière understand madness as a form of communication "in search of an echo" (p. 11). They foreground the idea that this "echo" might be found in the clinician, who, often through an uncanny shared history, comes to "hear" the message of the madness, thus registering it within time, history, and place. With a transpersonal understanding of enactment, this echo need not rely solely on a clinician in order to be witnessed but can also be realized within the fabric of our daily lives. The possibility then emerges that paranoid process might serve a healing function in and of itself. For this possibility to be realized, however, the echo madness seeks must somehow be found in terms of a synchronistic fit with the wider environment.

At the other end of the river where Anja lived was a long strip of beach dotted with cottages. The cottages were built in the 1920s and were intended for those afflicted with tuberculosis to convalesce. The structures were built by hand and were owned by the same families for multiple generations. Interestingly, while individual families owned the cottages, the land they resided on was government land. Although she was not a descendant of an original owner, Anja's paternal grandfather had lived in one of these cottages. He died from a medical complication when Anja was a small child, and her family inherited the house. Although Anja's childhood and adolescent years were largely unhappy, the cottage was a saving grace. Her family loved the cottage and some of her happiest memories took place there. Summers were spent with toes buried deep in the mud, searching for clams. Anja would spend hours marveling at the old wooden boards that comprised the ceiling, the stain of each plank imbedded with the perfect handprints of the original builders. As she daydreamed about these builder's lives, her mother would pick hundreds of beach plums and boil them down into sticky sweet jelly that was later spread on graham crackers. But, with conflict and hostilities increasing in her family, these idyllic hazy summer days became more and more punctuated by terror and violence. As Anja's heroin addiction progressed, she no longer spent time there; instead, she was thrown into the endlessly revolving door of hospital beds, twelve-step programs, psychiatrists' offices, methadone clinics, detox, and rehab. In 1995, a local bill began being pushed that would force the cottage owners to sign waivers which turned the rights of their cottages over to the government. Owners were allowed to stay in the cottages as long as they contributed to a fund that would later be used to demolish them.

The local bill regarding the cottages mobilized Anja's family into action. Anja's father became the makeshift leader of the resistance in opposing the government occupation of the cottages. Together with the other cottage owners, they launched a series of protests. Her father began unceasingly to research the history of the land, discovering it had precarious ownership – rumor had it that the land never was officially claimed by the US government and may have still belonged to the original Native American dwellers. The fight to keep their rights to the cottage banded her family together. They also became deeply connected to the wider cottage community, together that they had something worth fighting for.

Psychosis, alcoholism, and addiction can all be understood as related to extreme social disconnection. Unsurprisingly, there is a long-established connection between addiction and Indigenous peoples. In 1993, 75% of all Native American deaths were seen as directly or indirectly linked to alcohol use (Young, 1993). Anja and her father, both profoundly alienated, had each taken refuge in substances. However, as the campaign to save the cottages unfolded, the family found themselves more connected, both to others and also to the land. It was during this period that Anja's father stopped drinking and Anja herself successfully tapered off methadone.

Despite their best efforts, which spanned the course of several years, they were unable to save the cottages. The residents were forcibly removed, and on a cold winter's day in December, the government began demolition. Anja's family sat around the kitchen table, listening to the sounds down the river of the cottages being destroyed. For months afterwards, they all experienced the same reoccurring dream image – the cottage was still there, but they were no longer allowed entry. In the morning, they would tell each other these dreams and cry.

With reference to Sigmund Freud, Davoine and Gaudillière describe how dreams carry out the work of inscription – attempting to invoke in the dreamer the sense of anxiety, terror, or mourning that was left in a state of catastrophic suspension. Perhaps the dreams of Anja's family can be understood as transmissions from their Sámi ancestors. Ancestors, whose pain was now entering into history, finally allowing for the work of mourning to begin. This experience significantly shifted the dynamics within Anja's family, enabling them to become more vulnerable with each other and coinciding with an end to the years of domestic violence.

Conclusion

In keeping with the work of Davoine and Gaudillière, the shared familial delusion under consideration might be understood as pertaining to "pieces of history hitherto cut off from transmission" (p. 28). That is, the dispossession of Sámi people, both collectively and within Anja's family history, was a social catastrophe, one which led to the breaking down of social links. Never inscribed into time and place, the pain and fear of these ancestors presented itself generations later within her family as madness. Davoine and Gaudillière believe that the telos of "the symptom" is to find a person (i.e., a psychoanalyst) to "hear" its message. In the present example, we have sought to show that a transpersonal approach to enactment enables an understanding of the ways in which paranoid process can be inherently healing. This is expressed in terms of the striking series of external events which unfolded in meaningful coincidence with Anja's family history.

In the first place, there was the synchronicity of Anja's family coming to live on Native American land: the pushing up of arrowheads from the ground, the anthropology book documenting the lives of these Indigenous people, and, of course, the ghosts, all appear as part of a cosmic play, as though announcing a restoration of history and memory. Then, there is the uncanny fact that in conformity with the "delusion" regarding the DLA, the government did indeed take away the family home/land, this occurring in terms of the eventual demolition of the beach cottage. This synchronistic event can be understood as the "echo" the family were in search of and a historical repetition of Sámi history. In a further synchronicity, in 1995, the same year that the demolition of the cottages was set in motion, the Sámi people were first recognized as an Indigenous group by the Finnish government. The Constitution Act of Finland stated that the Sámi have a right to practice, protect, and strengthen their language and culture. Despite not providing the Sámi with formal rights to their homeland – which continues to this day to be owned by the Finnish government – this act allowed the Sámi to practice cultural autonomy within specifically sanctioned areas of Lapland. This meant that the Sámi were allowed to engage in the traditional customs of fishing and reindeer-herding, but that the land they resided on would not be theirs. The Sámi were permitted to use the land yet were not able to claim ownership of it, just as Anja's family were forced to sign over rites to the property upon which the beach house stood in order to maintain occupancy before the cottages were eventually torn down.

Critical psychologist Rachel Liebert (2018) reflects on the ways in which capitalism and colonization have only been made possible through the "de-supernatualizing" (p. 78) of being, and an ensuing "battle against magic" staged by the dominant Western hegemony (p. 139). Both of these tendencies alienate people from the earth, cosmos, animals, plants, spirits, God, and each other, thus creating the conditions needed for the proliferation of global capitalism. Liebert thus sees the medicalization of madness as evidence of a "war on imagination" which continues to perpetuate the rhetoric of colonization. She argues that the otherworldly nature of paranoia has a decolonizing potential, particularly in so far as it stands as a direct challenge to scientific discourse.

In the present chapter, we have focused on the teleology of paranoia so as to articulate a more emancipatory perspective on madness. This perspective has direct ties to practices within traditional Sámi culture. We find that in particular, the concept of *adjagas*, or the hypnogogic state between waking and dreaming, is congruent with a transpersonal perspective on enactment. With this in-between state of *adjagas*, the Sámi seek to reconnect with their land and ancestors by experiencing and communing with their essence (Kramvig, 2015). This essence or spirit can come in the form of memories, stories, or *joik*, which are spiritual songs that evoke a person or place. It is through the performance of these stories, memories, or *joik* that the individual can reconnect with their ancestral past. Kramvig (2015) offers the following example:

> When I got married, the ritual was held in a cave (named Kirkhelleren) on one of the many islands on the coast of Helgeland in Northern Norway. This is an area were local historians and local mimesis emphasize the cultural heritage as being Norwegian, although this view can be contested; archeology and history tell a different story and more complex story of the dynamic migration of Sámi and Norwegian settlements in the area. One of our friends attending the wedding was a young Sámi artist, and he was going to the cave for the first time. One night prior to arriving he had a dream in which he found himself in the cave. Dwelling within that landscape, a *joik* came before him. It was the voice of the place, the sense of the place, that came in the dream. He awoke with the *joik* still present. Kirkhelleren was announcing itself as real and came into the life of the person through the dream. When the artist arrived he brought his *joik* and performed it in our wedding cave. Therefore, the *joik* of the cave came back to the cave, and this reconnection brought the Sámi heritage into the present and into real existence, a presence that had been forgotten for a long time. After the event some of the people from the area came to him, fumbling but still talking about the sorrow of their own loss of connection with Sámi heritage, a heritage almost forgotten but one that was recalled by the event.
>
> (p. 191)

Kramvig (2015) concludes that contemporary Sámi decolonization practices are contingent on the act of recalling the interconnectedness of the past and the present (p. 202). In this light, the approach outlined in this chapter can be understood to serve the function of a metaphysical act of transformation. Herein, madness is seen as purposeful – an event through which people can meaningfully connect with the past, and through which the past becomes meaningfully alive in the present.

References

American Psychiatric Association. (2013). *Diagnostic and statistical manual of mental disorders* (5th ed.). Arlington, VA: Author.
Aron, L., & Atlas, G. (2015). Generative enactment: Memories from the future. *Psychoanalytic Dialogues, 25*(3), 309–324.

Davoine, F., & Gaudillière, J. (2004). *History beyond trauma*. New York: Other Press.

Ferrer, J. N. (2002). *Revisioning transpersonal theory: A participatory vision of human spirituality*. Albany, NY: SUNY Press.

Fraiberg, S., Adelson, E., & Shapiro, V. (1975). Ghosts in the nursery: A psychoanalytic approach to the problems of impaired infant-mother relationships. *Journal of American Academy of Child Psychiatry, 14*(3), 387–421.

Grof, C., & Grof, S. (2017). Spiritual emergency: The understanding and treatment of transpersonal crises. *International Journal of Transpersonal Studies, 36*(2), 30–43.

Harris, A., Kalb, M., & Klebanoff, S. (Eds.). (2016). *Ghosts in the consulting room: Echoes of trauma in psychoanalysis*. London & New York: Routledge.

Heisenberg, W. (1971). *Physics and beyond: Encounters and conversations*. London: G. Allen & Unwin.

Jung, C. G. (1952). Synchronicity: An acausal connecting principle. In *Collected works* (Vol. 8, pp. 417–531). Princeton, NJ: Princeton Universtiy Press.

Kramvig, B. (2015). Gift of dreams: Connecting to Sámi epistemic practice. In B. H. Miller (Ed.), *Idioms of Sámi health and healing*. Edmonton, Canada: The University of Alberta Press.

Laing, R. D. (1959/1965). *The divided self. An existential study in sanity and madness*. London: Tavistock. Reprinted, Harmondsworth: Penguin Putnam.

Liebert, R. J. (2018). *Psycurity: Colonialism, paranoia, and the war on imagination*. London & New York: Routledge.

Progoff, I. (1973). *Jung, synchronicity, and human destiny*. New York: Julian Press.

Slavin, M. O., & Kriegman, D. (1998). Why the analyst needs to change: Toward a theory of conflict, negotiation, and mutal influence in the therapeutic process. *Psychoanalytic Dialogues, 8*, 247–284.

von Franz, M.-L. (1980). *Projection and re-collection in jungian psychology: Reflections of the soul* (W. H. Kennedy, Trans.). La Salle & London: Open Court Publishing Company.

Weber, M. (1963). *The sociology of religion*. Boston, MA: Beacon Press.

Wexler, M. N. (1992). Psycho-social factors in shared family delusions. *International Journal of Sociology of the Family, 22*(1), 161–173.

Young, T. J. (1993). Alcoholism prevention among native-American youth. *Child Psychiatry and Human Development, 24*(1), 41–47.

Chapter 4

Re-turning the *Psykhe*

A creative experiment in decolonizing psychology[1]

Rachel Jane Liebert

ABSTRACT: Coloniality is a state of breathlessness. Elsewhere, I have argued that this suffocation is coiled through with paranoia, seeping into the cracks of white supremacy, stabilizing it. I call the force that animates these coils *psycurity*, and I consider how psycurity also moves through Psychology. However, paranoia's presence may also signal an otherworldly correspondence otherwise exiled within coloniality. This more-than-human capacity – what I come to call *imagination* – is twisted into paranoia within a context of fear, experiencing a kind of ontologic injustice. Yet, if these roots can be re-turned, perhaps they could offer something for decoloniality. In this chapter, I reflexively analyze a public art project to experiment with this idea. I come to wonder if practices of mystery, ritual, and pausing offer to fertilize, structure, and sustain a space for otherworldly correspondence within suffocating conditions. Obliging a compromise on what we Know, one to think/feel/act, and an art of immanent attention, these three practices can be approached as a tactic of *magical ideation* that offers psychologies fresh modes of *response-ability* when committing to decoloniality. This experiment therefore also experiments with re-turning the roots of our discipline – the study of *psykhe*, meaning both spirit and breath. Drawing attention to form over content, it asks: what if decolonizing psychology is a praxis of (not *on*) breathing?

KEY WORDS: art, decoloniality, imagination, more-than-human, psykhe

For Frantz Fanon (1952) – a founding and (conspicuously) forgotten figure of decolonizing psychology – colonization is the "worm-eaten roots" of society that need to be excavated and expelled (p. 4). Yet where there are worm-eaten roots, there are worms:

> We might imagine re-turning as a multiplicity of processes, such as the kinds earthworms revel in while helping to make compost or otherwise being busy at work and at play: turning the soil over and over – ingesting and excreting it, tunneling through it, burrowing, all means of aerating the soil, allowing oxygen in, opening it up and breathing new life into it.
>
> (Barad, 2014, p. 168)

This quote from queer theorist Karen Barad (2014) suggests that Fanon's worms might offer guidance for "re-turning" the roots of coloniality – the current-day presence of colonization, itself characterized by conditions of breathlessness (Maldonado-Torres, 2016).

Elsewhere, I suggest that such suffocation is coiled through with paranoia – a spiraling "desire-to-know" that grows within a context of fear and seeps into the cracks of white supremacy, stabilizing it. I call the force that animates this neocolonial security state *psycurity*, and I consider how it also moves through Psychology, a discipline with its own founding and (conspicuously) forgotten roots: the study of *psykhe*, meaning both spirit and breath. Indeed, my subsequent "reparative reading" (Sedgwick, 2003) of psycurity suggested that there may be more to paranoia than met my eye – that of a white critical psychologist, descended from settlers and trained and practicing in the global North.[2] With the help of a strange philosopher (see Stengers, 2011) and goddess (see Anzaldúa, 1987), I dug into the etymological roots of paranoia as *beside-the-mind* and came to wonder if the presence of paranoia signals a capacity for "otherworldly correspondence" – exiled within coloniality by what Sylvia Wynter (2003) has termed the "desupernaturalization" of our modes of being human. I call this more-than-human capacity *imagination* and argue that, twisted into paranoia, it experiences a kind of ontologic injustice within psycurity, within Psychology (Liebert, 2017, 2019).

Wynter (2003) too describes desupernaturalization as reinscribed through Science (in the singular and with a capital "S"; as discussed further in what follows) and, in turn, as possibly interrupted through the staging of encounters between Science and art. And so, inspired also by the co-incidence of Fanon and Barad previously described, in what follows I put my experience of a collaboration with a visual artist into proximity with worms to theorize re-turning the roots of paranoia as a means to theorize re-turning the roots of coloniality. More specifically, I take on a creative apprenticeship with paranoia vis-à-vis a measure of its potential known as magical ideation, to learn how one might make space for imagination within a neocolonial security state. Composting psycurity, my hope is that this experiment offers Psychology fresh modes of *response-ability* within contemporary conditions of breathlessness while calling attention to the importance of form as much as content when committing to a decolonizing praxis, when becoming a study of (not on) *psykhe*.[3]

Space-making

Over the past two decades, a transnational movement has been taking place within psychiatry to identify and intervene on young people who may *become* psychotic – a "mental illness" commonly associated with pathological paranoia. This state of potential (known as the "prodrome") is assessed via the Structured Interview for Psychosis-Risk Syndromes (SIPS; Miller et al., 2002) – an amalgamation of a number of different measures including magical ideation. Magical ideation is formally defined as "the belief, quasi-belief, or semi-serious entertainment of the possibility that events which, according to the causal concepts of this culture, cannot have a causal relation with each other, might somehow nevertheless do so" (Eckblad & Chapman, 1983, p. 215). To construct the first and most authoritative scale for magical ideation, Mark Eckblad and Loren Chapman (1983) drew on clinical case studies and psychoanalytic theory, drafting forty-two potential items and administering them to 227 undergraduates along with tests of acquiescence and social desirability, where those items that correlated too highly were made "more specific" or "less embarrassing," respectively. A revised scale was then given to two successive samples of undergraduates – 373 people in total – before being revised again to reach their final thirty true/false items, launching a trajectory of "pre-schizophrenic" research that led Loren Chapman and Jean Chapman, a decade later, to receive the American Psychological Association's Distinguished Scientific Award for the Applications of Psychology.

The reparative reading mentioned previously redirected attention to not just the liveliness of paranoia's potential but also its poisoned milieu, inviting an *apprenticeship* with paranoia, understood by Phillippe Pignarre and Isabelle Stengers (2011) as finding new ways of being efficacious by "learning the antidotes against what has been poisoned, and continues to poison, the situation" (p. 95). Such poison is the divide between Truth and Illusion incised during colonization and enacted in the magical ideation scale's determination of people's experiences as True or False. To take on an apprenticeship with paranoia is in part to learn how one might treat this incision. For Isabelle Stengers (2012), this requires *thinking by the milieu*. That is, to turn our gaze away from the truthiness of magical ideation, casting a judgment from a place of Knowing, and toward the conditions that welcome it, or not, or somewhat.

Unlike Eckblad and Chapman's (1983) definition of magical ideation, such an approach "would not dream of addressing others in terms of the 'beliefs' they entertain about a 'reality' to which scientists enjoy privileged access" (Stengers, 2012, p. 2). Indeed, Stengers (2012) places thinking by the milieu against the "scientific conquering 'view of the world,'" a colonizing Science (in the singular and with a capital "S") that appears "bent on translating everything that exists into objective, rational knowledge" (p. 2), throwing a think-net over the world, disciplining it, settling it. Instead, thinking by the milieu recognizes that milieu make demands of that which they are trying to represent – demands that will not necessarily be accepted. For example, in Eckblad and Chapman's (1983) previously mentioned process for developing the magical ideation scale, the high rates of "acquiescence" could be indicative of the experiences resonating with people (not simply their tendency toward suggestibility); the high rates of "social desirability" could be indicative of the experiences being shameful for people (not simply their tendency to give pleasing responses). The possibility of these interpretations forces attention to the milieu of magical ideation, to the ecological conditions that shut down these experiences, exposing them to ontologic injustice.

An experiment, then, can be less a test of the object of inquiry than of the milieu itself. In turn, Stengers (2011) calls for an *adventure of the sciences* (in the plural and with a small "s") that involves the "creation of a situation enabling what the scientists question to put their question at risk, to make the difference between relevant questions and unilaterally imposed ones" (p. 2). Within this "very particular creative art," objects of inquiry become "enrolled as a 'partner'" (p. 2), such that sciences become a craft of making spaces that animate our objects, allowing them to test our tests. Such questioning of the questioners is a key tactic in contemporary decolonizing movements, which are increasingly targeting institutions that make, claim, inflict Truth (Maldonado-Torres, 2016). Disobeying dichotomies of Knower and Known, delinking narratives of progress and civilization, Stengers' art form is thus perhaps also an opening for sciences to do "aestheSis" (with the unsettled "S"; Vázquez & Mignolo, 2013) – a praxis that not only "perceives the wound of coloniality hidden under the rhetoric of modernity" but "moves towards the healing, the recognition, the dignity of those aesthetic practices that have been written out of the canon of modern aestheTics" (n.p.).

Not only perceiving the wound of Truth and Illusion but moving toward witnessing a more-than-human vitality otherwise whitewashed within the colonial episteme, *Missed Connections* became a multimedia attempt at this kind of craft. I collaborated with visual artist Holli McEntegart[4] to undertake an apprenticeship with paranoia by turning to magical ideation, learning how psychologies (in the plural and with a small "p") might welcome paranoia's choked potentials. During December 2014, a first iteration was performed in the United States. Daily anonymous postings of magical ideation statements were placed on New York's Craigslist "Missed Connections" (a public website for realizing romantic and deviant fantasies), coupled with an email address for private responses, mapped to a physical location around New York City, scribed there in pencil, photographed, left to be rubbed off by elements or touch. Inspired by the US Department of Homeland Security's "anti-terror" slogan "If you see something, say something," physical locations were randomly chosen during my daily commutes, echoing a banal everyday suspicion. During October 2015, a second iteration was performed in Aotearoa/New Zealand. Daily anonymous postings of magical ideation statements were placed on Auckland's Craigslist "Missed Connections," coupled with an email address for private responses, mapped to a physical location around the city, scribed there with pencil, photographed, left to be rubbed off by elements or touch (Figures 1a, 1b, 2a, 2b). Inspired by the 1907 Tohunga Suppression Act,[5] physical locations were specifically chosen to echo dis-membered dreams.[6]

Spurred by a recurring picture in my head and a voice from Holli's gut, *Missed Connections* grew from a collision of imagination, more followed than directed. Moving between one of the older and one of the newer settler colonies of the British Empire, it soon obliged attention to the coloniality of the milieu, as well as to the constitutive role of space in the making of things. Both of which invoked Barad's (2007) onto-epistemology of "agential realism," which rests on a recognition that "*we are part of that nature that we seek to understand*" (p. 67, her emphasis). It follows that theorizing itself is not "a spectator sport of matching linguistic representation to preexisting things" (p. 54), so much as a material practice of

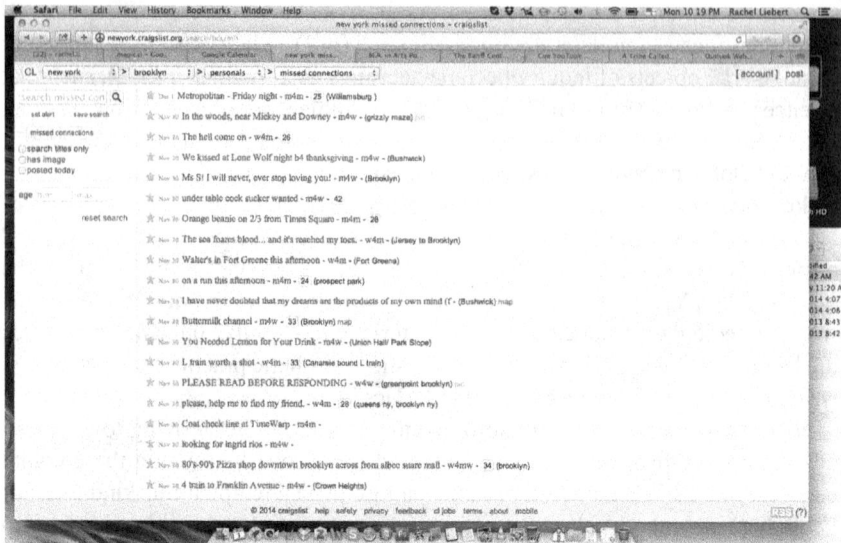

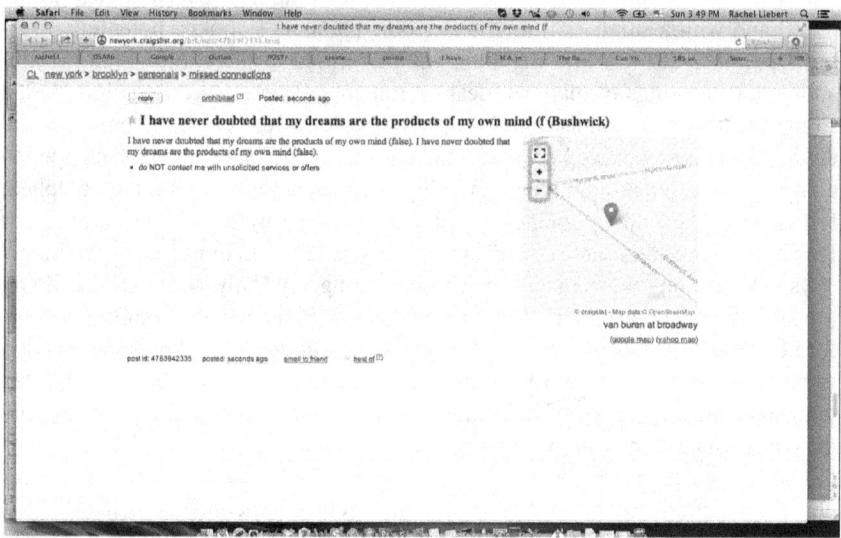

Figures 1a, 1b "Craigslist's Missed Connections"; *Missed Connections*, New York City, United States, 2015.

Source: Screenshot by Rachel Jane Liebert.

experimentation. Placing it beside Psychology, *Missed Connections* changed the context, the experimental apparatus, of magical ideation, helping me to think by the milieu, to theorize how space-making could be a mode of response-ability for

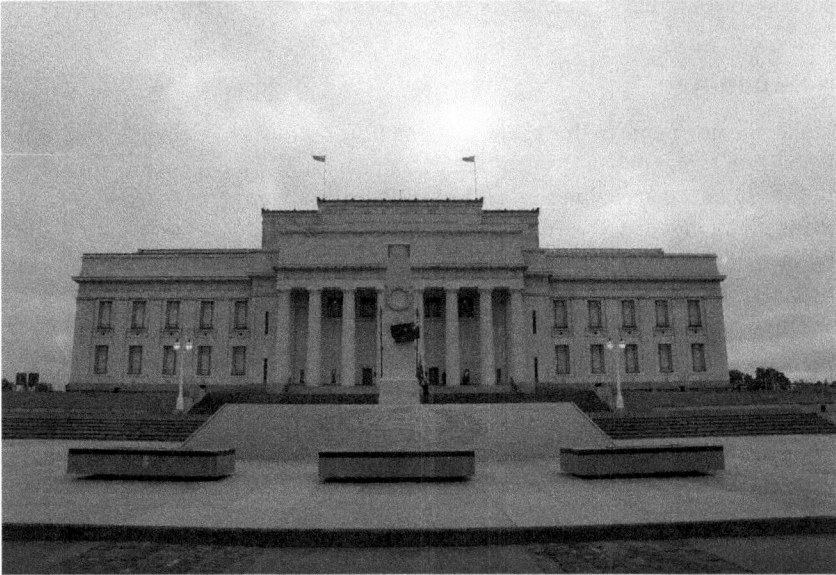

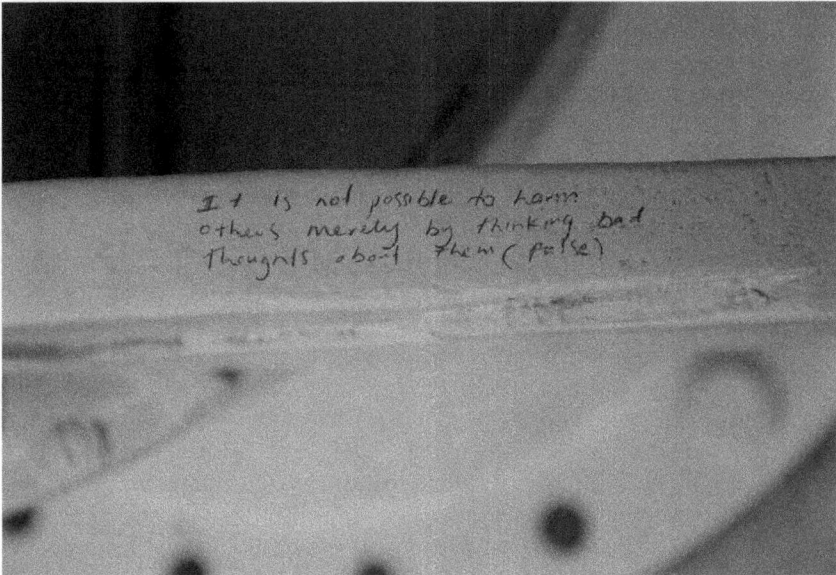

Figures 2a, 2b "It is not possible to harm others merely by thinking bad thoughts about them (false)," *Missed Connections*, Tāmaki Makaurau Auckland, Aotearoa New Zealand, 2015.

Source: Photo by Olivia Holmes.

psychologies seeking decoloniality. And thus to learn about not only re-turning paranoia's roots, but Psychology's – that breathless study of *psykhe* – too.

Re-turning

In the opening quote to this chapter, Barad (2014) enlists re-turning to talk about *diffraction* – "not only a lively affair, but one that troubles dichotomies" (p. 168). A sort of fractal reckoning of diffraction with itself, re-turning offers a spiraling methodology made up of *intra-actions*. Unlike relationships that are defined by interactions, presuming two or more pre-existing entities coming and acting together, intra-actions make things, enacting "agential cuts" that do not create absolute separations so much as "cut together-apart (one move)" (p. 168). Through intra-action, elements both come together and become separate, thus moving us away from the idea of "entities" and toward the idea of *entanglements*:

> Each bit of matter, each moment of time, each position in space is a multiplicity, a superposition/entanglement of (seemingly) disparate parts. Not a blending of separate parts or a blurring of boundaries, but in the thick web of its specificities, what is at issue is its unique material historialities and how they come to matter.
>
> (p. 176)

With diffraction, all phenomena (including supposedly disturbed perceptions) are entangled material agencies, a multiplicity of everything that is intra-acting to create them. Not creating unity, erasing difference – enacting difference, and turning our attention to how differences come to matter.

In turn, entanglements affect response-ability. For one, queering boundaries, they direct attention to otherness within – as happened in the previously mentioned reparative reading where paranoia was invited as a kind of "threshold phenomena" (Blackman, 2014), a "borderland" (Anzaldúa, 1987) vibrating with agential realism, with diffraction. As mentioned previously, this reading welcomed imagination – otherworldly correspondence – as part of paranoia's potential. In doing so, it pointed to the possibility of a "space of disjunct" within the coils of psycurity itself – that is, the potential to make something hopeful out of the fearful matter of paranoia (McManus, 2011). For Susan McManus (2011), one strategy for such "affective restructuring" might be turning technologies that are central to the production of fear against themselves; in this case, turning the tools that are used in psycurity back on psycurity, such that "fear is put to work in helpful ways" (n.p.).

In what follows, then, I attempt to articulate how one might re-turn paranoia's borderland soil, unearthing pockets of imagination. I attend to my experience of *Missed Connections* to turn paranoia's potential over and over again, reflexively musing on what the experiment's multiplicity of processes – its own ingesting/

excreting, tunneling, and burrowing – taught me about breathing new life into paranoia, and thus offered for psychological praxis within a neocolonial security state.

Ingesting/excreting: mystery

Ingest – *Transitive verb*: to take in for or as if for digestion

Excrete – *Transitive verb*: to separate and eliminate or discharge (waste) from the blood, tissues, or organs or from the active protoplasm

The craft of worms is in their digestion. With a mouth but no teeth, they take decaying matter in one end of their tubular bodies; break it down with moisture, micro-organisms, and muscle; absorb what they need; and release what is insoluble out the other end. It is these recycled "castings" that, containing nitrogen and other nutrients, nourish the soil, preparing the ground for new plant growth. If their tail is severed, they grow another, when they die, they digest each other. Hermaphrodites that can breed alone, there are over one million worms for every acre of land, said to have collectively digested every bit of fertile soil on earth. Underground, they are unseen to our eyes and un-needing of their own, although sensitive to light and touch. Eating waste and wasting food, death before life and life after death, both female and male, creating without vision, worms' ingesting/ excreting intra-acts the im/possible to fertilize conditions for something else.

Presenting an item on the magical ideation scale in a list (see Figure 1a), as a post (see Figure 1a), on the world (see Figures 2a, 2b), then switching to the next, *Missed Connections* was a montage, a series of fragments placed alongside one another. Escaping linear narrative or pregiven concepts or categories, it provoked curiosity, questions, meaning-making. It demanded participation. Yet the wide range of responses it solicited through Craigslist – flirting, anger, confusion, fear, censorship, silence – were given no answer. *Missed Connections* generated more questions. It released something lively. At the same time, having entered the world with no explanation, no mention, and indeed with no vision, *Missed Connections* required surrendering to not knowing where something was going, if anywhere – the posts disappeared from Craigslist after 45 days; the pencil disappeared from the world after rain, wind, snow, sea, touch. Too slippery to grip, the items of magical ideation were unknowable, obliging a multisensory groping in the dark, feeling (not seeing) the way. *Missed Connections* became about experimentation. Putting stuff out in public and seeing what happened. Including nothing. Riding my bicycle, re-cycling day after day, the experimentation of *Missed Connections* necessitated endurance, struggle. Continuing rain or shine or snow, it demanded the help of others. Passing things through, passing things along, bodies along, in order to pass the possibilities of magical ideation along. A kind of communal metabolism. Ingesting the magical ideation scale with no teeth, breaking it down into smaller pieces, and excreting something insoluble, ready for collective participation, *Missed Connections* fertilized conditions for something else.

Evoking a continual escaping, questioning, surrendering, experimenting, collectivizing, my experience with *Missed Connections* pointed me toward a practice of *mystery* for fertilizing spaces within psycurity. Contrary to being the antithesis of "hard science," mystery is stirring in contemporary approaches in neuroscience (e.g., Roy, 2016), botany (e.g., Myers, 2015) and physics (where mystery is "alive and well"; Barad, 2014), where – at least below the surface – it is breathing life into one's objects of inquiry, witnessing their vitality. Moreover, for Gabriel Marcel (1995), mystery brings a capacity to provoke an infinite line of questioning, thus shifting one's role away from figuring out The Answer – denying the dynamism of the world – to being an interlocutor. While not using the language of "mystery," Tobie Nathan (1999) similarly tasks psychologies to "always create fruitful material, open to elaboration, to new productions, to life" (n.p.) and has found it necessary to enlist a "contradictor" to do so – a partner or two or more that can help us question what we think and do, preventing us from biting down on it with the "big teeth" of "big concepts" (Pignarre & Stengers, 2011). In this context, "critique" is not an attack against which we defend theories and methods, so much as a form of collaboration to protect the liveliness of both practice and the world.

In turn, a problem is that which works to "gather together," not be (re)solved, and practice becomes a sort of "relay," "an itinerant definition of success, reinventing itself whenever a situation changes, assembling communities of new types of objectors (not sharing the same obligations)" (Pignarre & Stengers, 2011, p. 125). Rather than solutions, mystery invites responses in the form of trial and error, animating our response-ability with a commitment to collective experimentation. It thus perhaps offers psychologies a means to break the cycle of "epistemological violence" otherwise looming from the declarative authority of Science in our praxis (Teo, 2010). Indeed, compromising Knowing, mystery invites the presence of what Stengers (2012) calls "magic." While typically used to derogate efficacy, my experience with mystery suggested that this presence – etymologically deriving from *magh*, "to be able" – offers to capacitate psychologies. To admit magic is to surrender to not Knowing, to things not being Knowable; an admission necessary for imagination. Anzaldúa (1987), for example, considers her practice of writing – whether theory, story, or poetry – as an encounter with something more-than-human that first requires her to "let the walls fall down" (p. 97). These walls are those that demarcate the borders between worlds; Anzaldúa's surrendering guides her through/to otherworldly correspondence. Mystery offers to breathe new life into a space.

Intra-acting what is im/possible, mystery in turn enacts an indifference to colonial theorizing, to "piercing . . . through the sediments of psychological and epistemological 'depths'" (Trinh, 1989, p. 48). Here, Trinh Minh-ha (1989) is instead advocating for respecting the "realm of opaqueness" that comes with a "foreign thing"; an ongoing opacity that in turn generates conditions for an ongoing questioning – declared by Fanon (1952) as necessary for anticolonial revolution. Mystery thus enables a kind of decolonizing deference that perhaps also helps with "smelling the smoke," with feeling a discomfort from that present colonial past of hunting and burning, diagnosing and treating, as though we Know (Stengers, 2012). At the same time, approaching everyone as captured by this lineage, mystery allows for us to unashamedly need each other – setting the "bar of reason" as "not a privileged epistemic subject but an intersubjective community: the whole world" (Maldonado-Torres, 2006, p. 128). In this way, mystery also aligns with "border thinking," with choosing interlocutors who could open us to readings that lie beside a colonial episteme (Mignolo, 2012). Digesting the world in ways that are humble, participatory, and communal, mystery offers to metabolize the soil of paranoia, re-turning its roots within a neocolonial security state. In doing so, mystery could fertilize a space for otherworldly correspondence, for imagination, breathing new life into psycurity, into Psychology.

Tunneling: ritual

Tunneling – *Intransitive verb*: to make or use a tunnel

Tunnel – *Noun*: a horizontal passageway through or under an obstruction

The craft of worms is in their tunnels. Simple and segmented, their bodies move in a rhythmic pulse, shifting their front half forward, anchoring it with small hairs – "setae" – then pulling their back half to meet it. As they move in this way through the soil, they leave body-shaped tubes in their wake. At the same time, a mucus mixed with undigested soil is secreted out their ends, lining the tubes. Through this repetitive motion of wriggling and reinforcement, a network of enduring tunnels is built that provides drainage and aeration for the soil. And, when they die, they are digested by other worms – secreted as the reinforcing mucus, becoming the tunnel they were making, continually lubricating the flow of water and air, connecting past and future. Their bodies both molding and being tunnel, worms' tunneling intra-acts it/self to structure the conditions for something else.

With statements anonymously posted online and scribed onto physical surfaces, in *Missed Connections*, magical ideation came from the world (see Figures 2a, 2b). The "I"s becoming *both* its readers *and* something else – the more-than-human, worming its way into perception. Yet this otherworldly vitality was dependent on a movement between registers. Literally tethering the metaphysical and the physical, the virtual and the real, the human and the nonhuman, *Missed Connections* demanded a daily routine. A mundane rhythm of posting, cycling, scribing, photographing. Of posting, cycling, scribing, photographing. And repeat. The liveliness of magical ideation required constant tending, a pedaling, spiraling labor of maintenance conducted by my body – sometimes with joy, sometimes with anxiety, sometimes with nothing, but always something. Touching base on the regular.

Tunneling across worlds with mechanical movements, enacting a subterranean connectedness, *Missed Connections* directed an embodied approach for nourishing the more-than-human, structuring conditions for something else.

Simple, repeated, embodied, tending, my experience with *Missed Connections* pointed me toward a practice of *ritual* for structuring spaces within psycurity, witnessing and enacting a worldly involvement. For Stengers (2012), recovering this involvement means recovering a capacity to treat experiences as not "ours" so much as a beholding of something more-than-human, as "animating" us. Yet, locating subjectivity only in humans, Psychology creates a "unified front" against these experiences, thus first requiring a decentering of the human subject (Hillman, 1975). Nathan (1999), for example, approaches madness as "manufactured by things" – whether ideas, objects, operations, encounters – thereby redirecting his practice toward learning "to handle" these things, to "look after them, feed them, all the while receiving sustenance from them" (n.p.). Likewise for Anzaldúa (1987), witnessing a more-than-human vitality obliges treating it as having "the same needs as a person, it needs to be 'fed'" (p. 89). For her, such feeding happens through ritual – simple, repeated, embodied actions that give physical visible form to metaphysical invisible forces. Indeed, without ritual, something risks being, "a dead 'thing' separated from nature and, therefore, its power" (p. 90).

Ritual thus does not simply acknowledge the more-than-human, it enlivens it – opening possibilities for otherworldly correspondence, for imagination. For Hillman (1975), this openness is only possible if we also learn not how to make imagination our object so much as how to become *its* object, "giving over to the images and cultivating them for their sake" (p. 40). Not just watching and listening, but caretaking as they come and go. Ritual offers psychologies a way of taking care – an everyday labor that not only nourishes the more-than-human and our relationality, but also invites an experience of an agency that pulls "us" into being – that is, an experience of magic (Stengers, 2012), of "a force that obliges one to think/feel/act" (Pignarre & Stengers, 2011, p. 135). Crucially, such a practice can also involve words. At once able to capture, tame, and appropriate "the intangible as human" (Trinh, 1989, p. 53), words also make things matter (Barad, 2007) – a power well known by discursive psychologists, Indigenous peoples, and witches, and the opposite of the Western proverb, "Sticks and stones may break my bones, but words will never hurt me" (Elder, 2015). My experience with ritual suggested treating words – including those used in the magical ideation scale – as incantations. In turn, psychologies' diagnostics – whether of problems or people – can be seen as not determining *what is* so much as bringing into being a connection with *what else*. Ritual offers to breathe new life into a space.

Witnessing and enacting our worldly involvement, intra-acting it/self, ritual diffracts humanity across colonial borders, gently restoring an "ontological obliteration" central to the colonial project (Bhaba, 2004). Moreover its caretaking works as a kind of giving that, unlike the "imperial gift," animates the receiver (Maldonado-Torres, 2006); its embodiment works as a connective tissue that elevates the flesh, destabilizing the Cartesian hierarchy of capitalism, colonialism, and white supremacy; and its repetitiveness leaves a trace that joins time and space. All of which prevent a stuck-ness in one place or another, disturbing a linearity that is otherwise inhospitable to decolonizing possibilities (Rowe & Tuck, 2016). As Barad (2014), also drawing on Anzaldúa, writes, "tunneling through boundaries" is "not a bloodless but a necessary revolutionary political action)" (p. 175), for it is "not only that we live in many worlds at the same time, but also that these worlds are, in fact, all in the same place – the place each one of us is here and now" (p. 176). Clearing the airways between human and more-than-human, colonial and more-than-colonial, ritual offers to unblock the soil of paranoia, re-turning its roots within a neocolonial security state. In doing so, ritual could structure a space for otherworldly correspondence, for imagination, breathing new life into psycurity, into Psychology.

Burrowing: pausing

Burrow – *Noun*: a hole or excavation in the ground made by an animal (such as a rabbit) for shelter and habitation

Burrowing – *Intransitive verb*: to conceal oneself in or as if in a burrow

The craft of worms is in their burrows. Breathing through their moist skin, they struggle when things are too frozen, too hot, too bright – they become paralyzed if exposed to light for more than an hour. To evade these dry conditions, they dig down into the soil – up to 6 feet deep – and excavate a chamber with their bodies, lining it with a mucous to keep them moist, to help them breathe. To survive over prolonged periods, they use these burrows to curl into a tight ball, anchor themselves with their setae, and enter a reduced metabolic state – "aestivation" – waiting until the context becomes less suffocating. On the flip side, they will shift to overground when conditions are especially favorable – after rain or during high humidity – creating a mass movement that swiftly reaches new ground. Burrowing is also the means by which worms incubate their eggs, leaving them alone to survive even extreme weather until the babies sense it is safe to hatch and grow. Sheltering breath outside yet inside suffocating conditions, making a microcosm in order to make a macrocosm, worms' burrowing intra-acts the un/favorable to sustain conditions for something else.

By slipping magical ideation into not just Craigslist, but the beach, the construction site, the subway, the tourist spot, the strip-joint, the canon, the suburban street – *Missed Connections* excavated a space for the unexpected within the expected (see Figures 1a, 1b, 2a, 2b). Written in places of both reality and fantasy, both fear and desire, these statements could shelter outside yet inside a milieu that otherwise designated them as Normal or Psychotic, retaining their liveliness. Yet at the same time, the (true) or (false) billowing at the end of each statement suggested the casting of this dichotomizing, immobilizing light nearby. Sensing the dangers of judgment, *Missed Connections* invited digging down and staying in the darkness, waiting. Stretched over months, it adopted a regular but slow pace, nestling into the cracks of time and space yet paying attention, giving magical ideation a chance amidst suffocating conditions. Sustaining the conditions for something else.

Sheltering, sensing, waiting, slowing, attending my experience with *Missed Connections* pointed me toward a practice of *pausing* for sustaining spaces within psycurity. La Prieta – a character from Anzaldúa's short stories – suggests in an interview with Anzaldúa (n.d.) that she keeps falling through cracks because "it's dangerous to get too rigid and fixated on a certain kind of reality – that this reality is not all it appears to be. There are cracks in the picture," that "other worlds exist and they sometimes bleed into this one through the cracks" (p. 275). These cracks echo in what Stengers (2011) calls "interstices" – moments of more-than-human intrusion that suspend habits and solicit hesitation, a "precarious sense of the possible" (Pignarre & Stengers, 2011, p. 112). The power of these cracks is not in their revelation that there are cracks in the picture so much as in their revelation that the picture can crack. A practice of pausing, then, provides a refuge for this trembling sense, this gasp of air; interstices are not something that we make so much as shelter. Specifically, Stengers continues, they require a milieu that is protected from binaries. This kind of shelter is threatened within Psychology by everyday practices such as interpretation, which translates experiences into "ready-made theoretical tokens" (Nathan, 1999, n.p.). The challenge for psychologies is thus to not respond with a preconceived, overarching judgment, but to treat each experience as it comes, allowing its own immanent unfolding. That is, to give a chance – "the suspension of the probable, the holding out of a chance for the possible" (Pignarre & Stengers, 2011, p. 66). Pausing is perhaps a means to create this kind of breathing space, receptive to – and for – more-than-human intrusions, otherworldly correspondence.

For Anzaldúa (1986), another world "crops up when we least expect it" (p. 106) and "speaks to us in the moments when we are least aware" (p. 108). Again guided by Anzaldúa, Barad (2014) further writes that there "is no absolute outside; the outside is always already inside. In/determinacy is an always already opening up-to-come. In/determinacy is the surprise, the interruption, by the stranger (within) re-turning unannounced" (p. 178). Pausing may thus enable psychologies to make a space for these scholars' un/expected outside inside by taking on a kind of paradoxical vigilance – an "empiricism on alert" that aims to be caught off-guard, that is ready to be surprised (Stengers, 2011). In turn, pausing too invites an "art of immanent attention" to "what is good and what is toxic," to consequences rather than causes (Stengers, 2012, p. 8). My experience with pausing allowed for this kind of magic. Making a hole for imagination – Anzaldúa's (2002a) "la hoya" – it is a place where ideas can be "stirred and cooked to a new integration" (p. 292), creating microcosms for practicing and incubating another world. Pausing offers to breathe new life into a space.

Intra-acting the un/favorable, pausing makes a space not poisoned by a colonial lineage of this or that, casting a judgment as though we Know, but opening to a both/and. Far from idleness or apathy, it exemplifies the rigorous labor required of decolonizing work, where Maldonado-Torres (2016) describes "there is no place for laziness" (p. 11) – "Nothing can be automatically embraced as constructive and empowering; not everything can be rejected as a pure instrument of coloniality" (p. 11). Pausing appreciates that there is neocolonial in the decolonial and decolonial in the neocolonial. Encouraging a sharpened sensibility to shifty conditions, this "aesthetics of interruption" is particularly necessary within a colonial episteme built on ignorance (Watkins & Shulman, 2008). Indeed, it is perhaps an ally of what Anzaldúa (1993, 2002b) describes as "border art" – that which pokes holes in imposed worlds, allowing an "exten[sion] beyond the confines of our skin, situation, and condition" (p. 248). Making breathing space within suffocating conditions, incubating liveliness, creating microcosms, pausing offers to build shelters in the soil of paranoia, re-turning its roots within a neocolonial security state. In doing so, pausing could sustain a space for otherworldly correspondence, for imagination, breathing new life into psycurity, into Psychology.

Magical ideation

Fertilizing, structuring, and sustaining the space, putting my experience of *Missed Connections* into proximity with worms suggested that practices of mystery, ritual, and pausing may work together to turn the roots of paranoia over and over again, breathing new life into it. Allowing fresh air to come through ritual, be sheltered within pausing, and be metabolized through mystery, these three practices offer to make a space for otherworldly correspondence, for imagination, within suffocating conditions. Working from an agential realism that treats experiences as entanglements, the experiment diffracted the im/possible, it/self, and the un/favorable, directing attention to differences here-now and how these come to matter. In particular, given a context of psycurity, this composting opened a space for the decolonial in the neocolonial.[7] Mystery, ritual, and pausing thus offer a tactic for composting not only psycurity, but Psychology, too – reviving responseabilities for psychologies within a neocolonial security state.

Further, by respectively obliging a compromise on what we Know, one to think/feel/act, and an art of immanent attention, mystery, ritual, and pausing suggest *magic* might be a driving force behind such composting. For Stengers (2012), magic offers an antidote to our poisoned milieu for even the word itself "cannot be uttered . . . with impunity" (p. 134) – describing a craft as such warns of our descent from colonizers who violently desired, claimed to Know. Moreover, typically used as metaphor, "magic" resists capture, protecting practices from becoming yet another think-net. Mystery, ritual, and pausing can thus be thought of as a tactic for invoking magic-driven creation, a kind of *magical ideation* that makes a space for otherworldly correspondence. My experience of *Missed Connections* ultimately invited me to respond to psycurity, to the present political moment, by adopting an explicitly magical craft – a tactic that itself is lively enough to slip through the grip of Psychology, allowing psychologies to do a praxis that is *of* the imagination, not on it. Not disciplining, settling it; *making space for it*. Witnessing and welcoming a magic in the air that invites an experimentation here-now, such a tactic of magical ideation offers to not just compost but enchant the present (Pignarre & Stengers, 2011) – animating a response-ability both creative and militant in times of intensifying white supremacy, of breathlessness.

It is now two years since I first put my experience of *Missed Connections* into proximity with worms and learned about mystery, ritual, and pausing. Over this time, I have been testing out this tactic in my own psychological praxis of healing, pedagogy, and protest within a neocolonial security state. In these spaces, which I do not separate from one another, I have found a commitment to magical ideation increasingly useful. Mystery has helped me to respond to a demand for solutions used to refuse an engagement with problems, a lingering individualism, and assumptions that one does or should Know; ritual has helped me to respond to a tendency to prioritize cognition, an ignoring of the flesh and the more-than-human, a splintering of relationships, and a forgetting of what drives us from the past and from the future; pausing has helped me to respond to pressures for productivity, and to increasing trends toward being judgmental and exclusive that are otherwise undermining the safety of supposed "safe spaces." In turn, magical ideation has enabled me to make spaces that are both uncomfortable and generative, open to imagination, to that more-than-human, more-than-colonial correspondence that whispers another world is not only possible, but here-now. In conditions of intensifying white supremacy, with people feeling increasingly despondent or terrified, these modes of being human – both creative and militant – have felt at times like a breath of fresh air.

It is now another two years since I first wrote this piece, and – from where I stand in England (the germ of the British Empire) – calls for "decolonization" have become commonplace, including within Psychology. In particular this mainstreaming has manifested in university moves to "decolonize the curriculum"; moves that are being rolled out as more "diverse" content that is allowing yet further instantiations of colonial innocence, mastery, and arrogance (Tuck & Yang, 2012). In this stifling environment, I have found a tactic of magical ideation more useful than ever. Making a space for feeling feelings, pausing helps to interrupt innocence; making a space for ceding control, mystery helps to interrupt mastery; making a space for the more-than-human, ritual helps to decenter the human. However, most of all magical ideation has pointed me toward the importance of form as much – perhaps even more than – content when committing to decoloniality. While, its etymology suggests that Psychology is the study of *psykhe*, of spirit, of breath, our discipline was and is deeply implicated in the cosmological violence of coloniality, casting think-nets that smothered supernaturalized modes of being human, contributing to not just human but more-than-human genocide.

Instead of casting these think-nets even wider, what if we saw these roots as pointing to not our object of inquiry so much as our *mode*? What if "decolonizing Psychology" was a praxis *of* (not on) breathing? Making a space for listening to and collaborating with those who – and that which – know(s) that an-other world is not just possible and here-now but also urgently needed. Re-turning the *psykhe* of our studies and therefore our response-ability within coloniality, within a state of breathlessness.

Notes

1 This piece was originally published as "Compost" – one of seven chapters in *Psycurity: Colonialism, Paranoia, and the War on Imagination* (Liebert, 2019). It has been reprinted here with permission from Routledge as well as a revised introduction and conclusion, minor text edits, and some additional footnotes for clarity or context.

2 See footnote 5 for one way that this identity connects to my decolonizing praxis.

3 I try to write in a way that tries to enact my decolonizing commitments, including the tactic put forth in this piece, so my words and style may seem out of place in an academic collection premised on a colonial episteme-*cum*-institution. My hope is that readers might be able to sit with any discomfort that the form of this piece creates, trace the colonial contours of this discomfort, and listen for what whispers in its cracks.

4 Holli's praxis is in part guided by family lore – passed down by stories but unable to be "proven" – that her great grandmother was stolen as a child from her Indigenous family and raised as white by settlers. Nowadays referred to as "The Stolen Generation," this was an official, systematic program of kidnapping carried out by the Australian government under the British empire to erase indigeneity and complete the process of colonization.

5 Based on Britain's witch-hunting laws, the 1907 New Zealand Tohunga Suppression Act (TSA) criminalized tohunga – Indigenous healers rooted in relational ontologies that do not separate matter from spirit, mind from body, individual from world (Stewart-Harawira, 2005). After *Missed Connections* was completed, I found that my own ancestry is directly implicated in this cosmological violence. In 1864, my great-great-great grandfather was part of a setter militia who led a massacre against Rangiaowhia, a village designated as refuge for Māori elderly, women, and children during the war, and the main supplier of food for the anticolonial resistance. Eventually murdering 100 people, the militia began by surrounding a house with seven people inside, opening fire and then setting it alight. The people burned to death inside included the wife and two daughters of Kereopa Te Rau of the Ngati Rangiwewehi hapu of Te Arawa. Shortly thereafter, Te Rau became one of the original disciples and then leaders of Pai Marire – the first of a series of Māori spiritual movements committed to overthrowing settler dominance. Referred to as Hauhau – from "the breath of God" – the movement became known for its violent tactics, terrifying settlers, launching a government campaign of repression against Māori spiritualities that culminated in the TSA. Despite a liberal ruse of protecting Māori wellbeing, popular and judicial reports at the time explicitly show a desire to use the TSA to dismember the mobilizing, decolonizing capacities of tohunga (Voyce, 1989). And, as documented by Tūhoe psychologist Wiremu Woodard (2014), the TSA haunts contemporary mental health services in Aotearoa, where Indigenous healers and healing systems continue to be "suffocated and subjugated" (p. 41; see also Taitimu, Read, & McIntosh, 2018). For me, doing work within Psychology to interrupt this legacy is part of my present response-ability for my ancestor's past actions.

6 *Missed Connections* was subsequently installed in a gallery in Tamaki Makaurau Auckland and published in a book on more-than-human participation (see Brigstocke & Noorani, 2017). For more details, see www.magicalideations.com.

7 Worms, too. As I was looking into the practices of worms, I found a recurring claim, as exemplified in this extract from a *Journey North* website (https://journeynorth.org/search/WormNotes3.html#where): "Experts believe most native species were wiped out wherever glaciers covered the land. Most earthworms we see today were imported mainly from Europe by early settlers. The worms or worm cocoons traveled in the rootstocks of plants brought by the settlers from their homelands. Europeans added soil, with its earthworms or worm cocoons, to ships for ballast. Once anchored in North American harbors, ships released their ballast – and living worms, who found new homes." Depicted as intrepid pioneers, hard workers who tilled a soil already empty of inhabitants, it seems even worms come with a colonizing narrative.

References

Anzaldúa, G. (n.d.). A short Q&A between LP and her author (GEA). In A. Keating (Ed.), *The Gloria Anzaldúa reader*. Durham & London: Duke University Press.

Anzaldúa, G. (1986). Creativity and switching modes of consciousness. In A. Keating (Ed.), *The Gloria Anzaldúa reader*. Durham & London: Duke University Press.

Anzaldúa, G. (1987). *Borderlands La Frontera: The new Mestiza*. San Francisco: Aunt Lute Books.

Anzaldúa, G. (1993). Border arte. In A. Keating (Ed.), *The Gloria Anzaldúa reader*. Durham & London: Duke University Press.

Anzaldúa, G. (2002a). Speaking across the divide. In A. Keating (Ed.), *The Gloria Anzaldúa reader*. Durham & London: Duke University Press.

Anzaldúa, G. (2002b). (Un)natural bridges, (Un)safe spaces. In A. Keating (Ed.), *The Gloria Anzaldúa reader*. Durham & London: Duke University Press.

Barad, K. (2007). *Meeting the universe halfway*. Durham & London: Duke University Press.

Barad, K. (2014). Diffracting diffraction: Cutting together-apart. *Parallax, 20*(3), 168–187.

Bhaba, H. (2004). Framing Fanon. In F. Fanon (Ed.), *The wretched of the earth*. Paris: Presence Africaine.

Blackman, L. (2014). Immateriality, affectivity, experimentation: Queer science and future-psychology. *Transformations, 25*, 1–12.

Brigstocke, J., & Noorani, T. (2017). *Listening with non-human others*. Lewes: ARN Press. https://warwick.ac.uk/fac/soc/sociology/staff/blencowe/arn_press/listening_with_non-human_others_pdf.pdf. Last accessed March 9, 2018.

Eckblad, M., & Chapman, L. (1983). Magical ideation as an indicator of Schizotypy. *Journal of Consulting and Clinical Psychology, 51*(2), 215–225.

Elder, H. (2015). Te waka oranga: Bringing indigenous knowledge forward. In *Rethinking rehabilitation: Theory and practice* (pp. 227–246).

Fanon, F. (1952). *Black skin, white masks*. Paris: Editions du Seuil.

Hillman, J. (1975). *Re-visioning psychology*. Harper & Row.

Liebert, R. J. (2017). Beside-the-mind: An unsettling, reparative reading of paranoia. *Subjectivity, 10*(1), 123–145.

Liebert, R. J. (2019). *Psycurity: Colonialism, paranoia, and the war on imagination*. London & New York: Routledge.

Maldonado-Torres, N. (2006). Cesaire's gift and the decolonial turn. *Radical Philosophy Review, 9*(2), 111–138.

Maldonado-Torres, N. (2016). *Outline of ten theses on coloniality and decoloniality.* Frantz Fanon Foundation. http://frantzfanonfoundation-fondationfrantzfanon.com/IMG/pdf/maldonado-torres_outline_of_ten_theses-10.23.16_.pdf. Last accessed March 9, 2018.

Marcel, G. (1995). *The philosophy of existentialism* (M. Harari, Ed.). New York: Carol Publishing Group.

McManus, S. (2011). Hope, fear, and the politics of affective agency. *Theory and Event, 14*(4).

Mignolo, W. D. (2012). *Local histories/global designs: Coloniality, subaltern knowledges, and border thinking.* Princeton, NJ: Princeton University Press.

Miller, T. J., McGlashan, T. H., Rosen, J. L., Somjee, L., Marcovich, P. J., Stein, K., & Woods, S. W. (2002). Prospective diagnosis of the initial prodrome for schizophrenia based on the structured interview for prodromal syndromes: Preliminary evidence of interrater reliability and predictive validity. *American Journal of Psychiatry, 159,* 863–865.

Myers, N. (2015). Conversations on plant sensing: Notes from the field. *Natureculture, 3,* 35–66.

Nathan, T. (1999). *Georges Devereux and clinical Ethnopsychiatry* (C. Grandsard, Trans.). Paris: Centre Georges Devereux. www.ethnopsychiatrie.net/GDengl.htm. Last accessed March 9, 2018.

Pignarre, P., & Stengers, I. (2011). *Capitalist sorcery: Breaking the spell* (A. Goffey, Trans.). London: Palgrave Macmillan.

Rowe, A. C., & Tuck, E. (2016, June). Settler colonialism and cultural studies: Ongoing settlement, cultural production, and resistance. *Cultural Studies Critical Methodologies,* 1–11.

Roy, D. (2016). Neuroscience and feminist theory: A new directions essay. *Signs: Journal of Women and Culture in Society, 41*(3), 531–552.

Sedgwick, E. (2003). *Touching feeling: Affect, pedagogy, performativity.* Berkeley: Duke University Press.

Stengers, I. (2011). *Thinking with whitehead: A free and wild creation of ideas.* Boston, MA: Harvard University Press.

Stengers, I. (2012, July). Reclaiming animism. *e-flux Journal, 36,* 1–10.

Stewart-Harawira, M. (2005). *The new imperial order: Indigenous responses to globalization.* Wellington, NZ: Zed Books.

Taitimu, M., Read, J., & McIntosh, T. (2018). Nga Whakawhitinga (standing at the crossroads): How Maori understand what Western psychiatry calls 'schizophrenia'. *Transcultural Psychiatry,* 1–25.

Teo, T. (2010). What is epistemological violence in the empirical social sciences? *Social and Personality Psychology Compass, 4*(5), 295–303.

Trinh, M. (1989). *Woman, native, other: Writing postcoloniality and feminism.* Bloomington & Indianapolis: Indiana University Press.

Tuck, E., & Yang, W. (2012). Decolonization is not a metaphor. *Decolonization: Indigeneity, Education & Society, 1*(1), 1–40.

Vázquez, R., & Mignolo, W. (2013). Decolonial AestheSis: Colonial wounds/decolonial healings. *Social Text Online.* https://socialtextjournal.org/periscope_article/decolonial-aesthesis-colonial-woundsdecolonial-healings/. Last accessed March 9, 2018.

Voyce, M. (1989). Māori healers in New Zealand: The Tohunga suppression act 1907. *Oceania*, *60*(2), 99–123.

Watkins, M., & Shulman, H. (2008). *Toward psychologies of liberation*. New York: Palgrave Macmillan.

Woodard, W. (2014). Politics, psychotherapy, and the 1907 Tohunga suppression act. *Psychotherapy and Politics International*, *12*(1), 39–48.

Wynter, S. (2003). Unsettling the coloniality of being/power/truth/freedom: Towards the human. *The New Centennial Review*, *3*(3), 257–337.

Chapter 5

Divine madness
Exceedance and not-knowing

John Gale

ABSTRACT: In the *Phaedrus*, Plato speaks of various forms of madness having a divine origin, and bestowing virtue on mankind. A similar, though not equivalent, elevation of madness over sanity is found in the Pauline epistles, where Christians are described as fools. Diogenes of Sinope and a number of other Cynics, as well as Christian ascetics, adopted a way of life that could reasonably be described as mad. This challenged received ideas about sanity, and in so doing, emphasized its social aspect. The prophet and the poet were seen in antiquity to disclosed truth, in enigmatic sayings and in odd turns of phrase that stretch everyday usage. This overstepping of reason (logos) links both inspired madness and simulated madness to the lexis of mysticism. They are, in other words, a stance, in relation to knowing, that is shared by philosophy. To use Heidegger's idiom, the latter is nothing other than a rambling path through the forest, one which often leads nowhere. But sometimes comes to a clearing in which Being itself is made manifest as *ek-stasis*.

KEYWORDS: ecstasy, Freud, Heidegger, madness, Plato, *Apophthegmata Patrum*

Even without a complete collocation of the lexicon of madness in Greek literature, it is clear that in antiquity, madness was not always seen in a negative light. Indeed, in a celebrated passage in the *Phaedrus*, Plato, the "father of psychoanalysis," says that it is not an evil, nor is it shameful or disgraceful.[1] Rather, certain of its manifestations are of divine origin, superior to sanity and the source of our greatest blessings. Thus, he says, the poetry of a sane man vanishes into nothingness before that of the inspired madman.[2] Furthermore, Plato thought that the prophetess at Delphi and the priestesses at Dodona and the Sibyl conferred many splendid benefits upon Greece when they were mad but few when they were in their right minds. Indeed, "for him who is possessed of madness a release from present ills is found" and he is safe (Plat. Phaed. 244a–e). It may not be insignificant in this regard that in the *Theaetetus*, Socrates says that people describe him as *atopōtatos* – out of place, strange, absurd, disconcerting – and his work, an *aporia*, a puzzle (Plat. Theaet. 149a).[3] Alcibiades stresses the point by describing

Socrates as someone who evades classification, a misfit who does not conform to any common type of personality (Plat. Symp. 221c–d; cf. Hadot, 1987). Consequently, he was, as Diogenes Laertius pointed out, someone "despised and laughed at" (DL 2.21).

Foolish wisdom

Something similar is found in the Pauline corpus where Christian belief is described as a form of madness and believers, fools (*mōroi*[4]). Once again, it is a divine madness: "let him become a fool (*mōros genesthō*) that he may be wise" (1 Cor. 3.18). This is particularly interesting. Not only does it contradict things Paul says elsewhere – e.g. when accused of being mad, he replies, "I am not mad (*ou mainomai*), rather I speak words of sober truth" (Acts 26.25) – but it also reverses the meaning of *mōros*, as we find it both in its verbal form in the synoptics and in the tradition of the sayings of Jesus, the latter of which broadly fall within the parameters of Old Testament usage (Welborn, 2005).[5] One possible source, according to Gibb (1941), is the logion in which the "wise and learned" (*sophōn kai sunetōn*) from whom things are hidden, are contrasted with the babes (*nēpiois*) to whom they are revealed (Matt. 11.25/Lk. 10.21). But it is also possible that Paul had in mind the Cynics, a number of whom, as Diogenes of Sinope, one of the founders of Cynicism, behaved in a very unconventional way, farting, defecating and masturbating in public and generally being socially disruptive (DL VI. 2 passim).[6] Plato famously described him as "a Socrates gone mad (*mainomenos*)" (DL VI. 54). Fundamental to Cynicism was the idea that doctrine should not be separated from the manner in which a philosopher lived. It was not enough to criticize social conventions and established values; the philosopher had to express this in the way he behaved and in his appearance. Because of this focus on ethics rather than logic and physics, some thought Cynicism not really a philosophy at all, but merely a way of life (*enstasin biou*) (DL VI. 103). Yet it was for this very reason that Pierre Hadot (1987) considered Cynicism fell within the tradition of philosophy as a spiritual exercise (*askēsis*). It was a gradual, lifelong conversion (*epistrophē*) that brought a person to critique received ideas, including what it meant to be sane or insane. Importantly, the Cynic philosopher refused to identify himself as a sage. In this we can see Cynicism coming far closer to the apophatic tradition of not-knowing than we might at first expect.[7] *Apophasis*, a concept central to mystical discourse, refers to an affirmation of an absence of knowledge about the divinity. Underlying this is the notion that the divinity is beyond being, and thus beyond language or mind. To use Wittgenstein's idiom, it is an understanding that there are things which are "not a part of the world" – and are consequently unknowable (T. 5.641).[8] Nevertheless, although outside the symbolic (Lacan), the realm of the unsayable (the mystical) nonetheless exists. Thus, Heidegger writes that "even the nothing . . . in the sense that it is thought or spoken 'is' something" (Heidegger, 1959, p. 40).[9] It is this paradox, moreover,

that led pseudo Denys to assert that not-knowing or unknowing (*agnōsia*) sur-
passes knowing, as the latter is always an inaccurate means of expression (Lossky,
1957).[10] Or as it is expressed in the Socratic paradox "I am wiser . . . as I do not
know anything" (Plat. Apol. 21d).[11]

Simulated madness

We can distinguish two schools within Cynicism; one ascetic, the other mystical
(Oltramare, 1927 cited in Attridge, 1976, p. 17. n 33). Aspects of both schools
passed over into Christianity,[12] and we find Origen (C. Cels. 2. 41) and Basil (Ep.
4) praising the Cynic way of life. This carrying over is particularly evident in
the monastic tradition (Goulet-Cazé, 1986). There are examples of monks behaving in an intentionally provocative and anti-social way in the *Apophthegmata
Patrum*.[13] These are collections of oral anecdotes from the 4th and 5th centuries
(Bousset, 1923),[14] redacted in the sixth, from the Egyptian monastic centers of
Nitria and Scetis (Špidlík, 1963). Here, in a kind of reversal, Abba Antony is
reported to have said that a time was coming when men will go mad, and when
they see someone who is not mad, they will say: "You are mad (*mainē*), you are
not like us" (Apoph. Pat. Antony 25). This element of difference or otherness permeates the discourse of madness through the ages. Guillaumont (1996) has argued
that madness was assumed by Christian monks as a form of withdrawal from the
world (*anachorēsis*), which was a key aspect of *askēsis*. *Askēsis* referred not just
to physical training in endurance, but to an interior work (*to ergon tēs psuchēs*)
(Apoph. Pat. Theodore of Pherme 10, 11).[15] This notion, fundamentally Cynic,
was probably transmitted to the Church Fathers via Philo, who was instrumental
in developing the notion that mystical experience was a kind of "sane madness"
(*sōphrōn mania*) (Dudley, 1937).[16] When people came to see him, it was said of
abba Ammonas that he used to feign madness. "A woman standing near him said
to her neighbour, 'The old man is mad.' Abba Ammonas heard it, called her, and
said, 'How much labour have I given myself in the desert to acquire this folly'"
(Apoph. Pat. Ammonas 9).[17] A number of other desert fathers were called fools
(e.g. Apoph. Pat. Moses 8). Palladius describes a nun in the monastery at Taben-
nisi who was *salos* (Pall. h. Laus. 34: 3–7),[18] a word that can mean imbecile, half-
witted, a fool, or mad (Lampe, 1961, p. 1222). Although its etymology is obscure,
Špidlík suggested it may come from the Syriac *sakla* because of its use in the
Peshitta to translate the Greek *mōroi*.[19]

The tradition of "fools for Christ," as they became known, continued into the
Byzantine period. In the 6th century, John Rufus describes a monk in Silvanus's
monastery near Eleutheropolis in lower Egypt, who pretended to be mad (*prospoi-
umenos mōrian*). He laughed when others came near him. When three visitors
came to the monastery and asked to see all the monks, Silvanus told them not to
try to see the mad one (*salos*)[20] because he would scandalize them. However, they
demanded to see him and found him in his cell, where he was putting pebbles into

two baskets. He answered their questions by laughing at them (Pleroph. 178–179). We find examples of other ascetics walking around naked, living on the streets, behaving disruptively and saying strange impenetrable things. The 7th-century life of Symeon the Fool by Leontius of Neapolis (Festugière, 1974) is probably based on that of Diogenes of Sinope (Rydén, 1963). It depicts the saint dancing licentiously with prostitutes, gorging himself on cakes during a period of fasting, and defecating and farting in public. His intention may have been prophetic, in the sense that by his behavior, Symeon aimed at challenging what he saw as hypocritical distinctions between what was acceptable and unacceptable, sane and insane. In so doing, he confronted false self-knowledge, a knowledge based on the ego, and realized what Lacan calls *savoir* (which he distinguishes from *connaissance*), a genuine form of self-knowledge, which is simultaneously a not-knowing.[21] Later, this tradition of foolishness is translated into a Russian idiom (*yurodivy*) and continued there well into the 19th century, and we find it famously referenced in characters in novels by Pushkin, Dostoyevsky, and Tolstoy.

Yet, although a prophetic element may have been intended, we should not lose sight of the fact that this madness was artificial, a pretense[22]. Despite the clear similarities, Cynic philosophers and Christian monks chose to adopt a subversive and unconventional "mad" lifestyle. They acted as if they were mad. This radically separates these traditions of "foolishness" from the divine madness of which Plato spoke.[23] The latter was, above all else, something that happened to a man. Madness seized him, fell upon him, "without him choosing it or knowing why" (Dodds, 1959, p. 218). This latter kind of madness functioned in the way grace functioned in religious discourse. Nevertheless, there was still present in the faux madness of the Cynic philosopher and the Christian ascetic, a belief that their madness would bear fruit in the form of certain "blessings" the most notable of which was *apatheia* (impassivity; the disappearance of *pathē*). This ideal described a state of mind, which comes with a wisdom not disturbed by the passions.[24]

Inspired madness

While in Socrates' first speech in the *Phaedrus* (Phaed. 237a–241d), madness is opposed to *nous* (intelligence; awareness; intuitive intellect) and *sophrosyne* (soundness of mind; temperance), the antithesis is maintained in the second (244a–257b). Here, Socrates praises madness as infinitely superior to rationality (North, 2019). He identifies four forms of divine or positive madness – prophetic madness, telestic or ritual madness, poetic madness, and erotic madness. Each is inspired by its own god – Apollo, Dionysus, the Muses and Aphrodite. By describing some forms of madness as a gift of the gods, Plato is at once implying that there are other, forms of madness, the origins of which are physical rather than inspired.[25] What distinguished the two kinds, is that divine madness is always a cause of good.

The most important of the mysteries were those of Demeter and Persephone at Eleusis. The cult of Dionysus, god of wine, which we read about in Euripides, certainly involved ecstatic dancing and wine induced trance (Linforth, 1946b). This was probably the prototype of telestic, orgiastic madness. Dionysus is represented in Greek literature and in myth as an outsider, and women and slaves were prominent in the cult which brought about "mad" states through disinhibition in which a casting off of the ego seem to have allowed some kind of temporary social emancipation and catharsis (Dodds, 1959). Such cultic "letting go" may have served a social function of releasing irrational impulses that might otherwise have come out in more destructive forms. Above all, ritual madness was directed toward a cure.[26]

Erōs and an exceedance of language

It is clear from Aristotle that unlike many of the hypostatizations that appear in the early cosmogonies, Eros is not so much a state but a force (Met. 1071b). Sexual love is raised to the cosmological level. This is still in evidence in Plato's extensive treatment of love in the *Symposium*. Here, we find Socrates portrayed as a figure of Eros and as such transformed into an ideal (Patzer, 1987). Yet at the same time, Socrates, who proclaims "I know nothing, save about *erōs*" (Plat. Theag. 128b), functions as a mediator between a transcendent ideal of wisdom and human reality (Hadot, 1987).[27] In the *Lysis* and in the *Symposium*, he describes love as a consequence of desire (*epithumia*) and directed toward filling a lack (*endeia*; Symp. 200e–201b). As divine madness (*theia mania*), *erōs* is necessarily spiritual in the sense that it is concerned with the soul (*psuchē*) as well as with the body.[28] In this it brings a unity to man as he is in his bodily, sexual self and in his desire for transcendence. It involves an idealization of the beloved which suggests that the object of love is not exactly the visible reality of the beloved but the invisible or divine. The real object of desire is another reality of which the beloved is merely an image or reflection (Plat. Phaed. 249c). Here, divine *erōs* contrasts with an erotic love that is restricted to the visible beauty of the body. The latter may become a delirium but that would, in Plato's terms, be a human form of madness rather than a divine madness. The result of desire without regulation (Plat. Phil. 63c. 45e, 47c).[29]

As we have seen, in the *Phaedrus*, Plato counted poetic ecstasy as one of the effects of divine madness.[30] "Possession by the Muses, and their madness, invade . . . [the] psyche, awaken it, and bewitch it with . . . poetry; and by glorifying countless deeds of our forefathers, educate posterity" (Plat. Phaed. 245a). Although Plato developed this view, it was by no means uniquely his.[31] Indeed, the words gathered up by the poet seemed to many in antiquity to have their source elsewhere. Plato had inherited it from the pre-Socratic philosophers, particularly Heraclitus and Empedocles (Delatte, 1934).[32] Democritus held that the finest poems were written with inspiration and a holy breath (*enthousiasmou kai hierou pneumatos*) (Billault, 2002). Later, Cicero refers to the poet as holy precisely because his words are divinely inspired.[33] This was surely nothing other than a reaction to the utter profundity of the poet's verse, which suggested to the listeners that the source of the poetic *logos* lay beyond the imaginary or specular (Lacan, 2006). Beyond the ego. In its earliest form, the poet is seen merely as the messenger of the Muses (see Plat. Theag. 769). But this intuition deepens in the transition that has already taken place by Plato's time, where the Muse is thought to be actually inside the poet (Plat. Crat. 428c).

This way of thinking is not too dissimilar to the early modern understanding of mystical verse, in which the poet feels he has been taken out of himself in rapture. An outstanding example of this is found in the work of the 16th century Spanish Carmelite, John of the Cross (Campbell, 1972). Like other mystics, he adopts an erotic vocabulary to speak of ecstasy.[34] Lacan considered that the poetry of John of the Cross was able to open up another dimension of experience to the reader, of which he was not conscious. This gave it, he thought, an authentically religious "tone" (*l'accent*) (Lacan, 1993, p. 77).[35] The notion that the poem might open up another dimension of experience is reminiscent of what Heidegger referred to as disclosure (*Erschlossenheit*), in which new horizons of meaning are laid open. Disclosure is a concept that Heidegger develops in 1927, in his unfinished magnum opus *Sein und Zeit*, in relation to a particular understanding of *alētheia* (truth) (SZ 33). Truth here does not refer to the acquisition of factual knowledge but an opening in intelligibility. A manner of speaking about the way in which being, previously concealed, is unfolded. After the Second World War, turning increasingly to questions of language in its manifold forms, and particularly poetry – largely represented by the work of Hölderlin and Rilke[36] – Heidegger wrote that it is only when the poet risks being mad, that he can he hear the message of being and disclose it (Tsai, 2018).[37] This, he considers, is an everyday process but not one that is accomplished through reason. Rather, it is the event of transcending oneself and the world. In fact, Heidegger describes the self and being-in-the-world as somehow brought together in such a way that being appears as their unique unfolding, as "the *transcendens* pure and simple" (Schürmann, 2008, p. 93). He says this points back to the ontological principle in Parmenides where, incidentally, it is set out within a poem.[38] Following Aristotle, Thomas Aquinas developed this idea.

> Thomas is engaged in the task of deriving "*transcendentia*" – those characteristics of Being which lie beyond every possible way in which an entity may be classified as coming under some generic kind of subject-matter (every *modus specialis entis*), and which belong necessarily to anything, whatever it may be. Thomas has to demonstrate that the *verum* is such a *transcendens*.
> (SZ 14)[39]

To refer to the self in this way is to be reminded that we cannot speak coherently about the self in terms of a person's pregiven inner states or subjective or spiritual apparatus, but only as a task yet to be achieved (SZ 115, 117). That is to say, the self must be understood as already engaged in a world, in relation to being-there (Dasein) and thus in relation to others.

Everdayness (*Alltäglichkeit*), does not refer to the surface of things in the sense of what is superficial, as Section 27 of *Sein und Zeit* shows (SZ 126). Gadamer, in relation to Celan, also argues explicitly in favor of the everdayness of poetry. "The 'hidden' language that the poet brings out into the open," he says, "is not anything occult, subterranean, or otherworldly . . . It is only the quotidian speech of ordinary mortals, language in all its human facticity, the word in everyone's mouth." (Gadamer, 1997, p. 5). In other words, a poem can be made of anything. "It doesn't have to be 'poetical' to be poetic" (ibid). In the course of some very dense arguments, Heidegger demonstrates that the reason why the subject encounters himself in everyday existence is precisely because that existence is prescribed by others. This emphasis on the everyday correlates, to some extent, with Lacan's description of the unconscious as outside rather than interior or deep, because it is linguistic and therefore intersubjective. Indeed, it is part of the everyday, as the exteriority of the symbolic in relation to man (Lacan, 2006, p. 469).

Yet while Plato described the poet as mad, in the sense that he is inspired by the Muses, he also established an inseparable connection between the poetic, *paideia* (education, culture) and *aretē* (virtue) (Jaeger, 1973, p. 428 n. 12). For in the classical understanding of poetry, the ethical or educative dimension was dominant and was only later displaced – principally by Christian authors – by an aesthetic view. In other words, what made a good poem in the ancient world was the effect it had on educating society and generating virtue, rather than how beautiful it sounded. This ethical dimension binds poetic discourse and the poet himself to tradition, in its original sense of a handing on (*paradosis*), within a discourse addressed to a specific community. For while the inspired word comes from a private, secret place, a poem is not a hermetic, sealed-off discourse. In other words, poetry is still language and therefore, however ambiguous or obscure it may be, a poem is not gibberish or nonsense but something intelligible, for the poet constructs and brings to birth a world that is dependent on the community from which he himself has received language.

However, although a poem uses words, it alters our relationship to language by stretching everyday usage. It demands a suspension of known terms – including the term poetry itself. Furthermore, our associations force us beyond the sense the poet intends, as he does not have the power to completely fix the meaning of a word from the flow of everyday usage (Lang, 1997). As the navel in Sigmund Freud's dream, there is always a part of the poem to which we remain deaf, not because we have not yet worked it out, but because it is too close an intimation of the mystical, of what is outside language. That is to say, the text becomes, in some sense, an absurdity because, by pointing beyond itself, it touches on that to which remains unsaid (T 6. 45). For this reason, we can say that madness signifies something essential in all poetic utterance. Namely, the fact that speech is always talking about something that is not manifest (SZ 32).

Prophecy and ecstasy

Twice in *Ion* (553d–536d) Plato refers to the frenzied dancing of corybantic possession as an analogy of poetic inspiration (*enthousiasmos*) (Linforth, 1946a).[40] Philo says that aided by music the devotees lose consciousness of everything. A belief in prophecy and divination (*mantikē*) was common in antiquity (Murray, 1912). And the figures of the prophet (*theios mantis*) and seers – "spokesmen of the supernatural" (Dodds, 1965, p. 53 n. 2) – occupied an important place in ancient Greece, and were both institutional and peripatetic (Fascher, 1927).[41] They were distinct from those who learned how to read the future from natural phenomenon, like the behavior of birds (augury) or the entrails of animals. Often, the seer functioned as a dissident, criticizing politicians and being critical of the status quo. Seers could see the truth and declaim it but were not able to enforce change. In this sense, although they were always right, they were, at the same time, powerless. They spoke enigmatically, and thus their messages needed interpretation, and we find a number of examples of conflicting interpretations. They were powerless, despite being in possession of a truth that they received from elsewhere. Here, in respect to prophecy, madness is a way of speaking about how to access a truth as yet unknown. This truth mostly concerned knowledge about the future. Indeed, the oracular is one of the things that distinguishes the prophet from his audience, which can only really speak about the past by drawing on memory. Thus, Foucault categorizes prophecy as a form of *parrhēsia* or "truth-telling," thus linking it to the tradition of spiritual exercises or *askēsis* (Foucault, 2014, p. 38). Often this foretelling presented, in the form of a riddle, a choice about the future direction the recipients can take in their lives.

Ecstasy, temporality, and thinking

As Dodds pointed out, the Greek word *ekstasis* and its cognates have a very wide range of applications including a state of awe or stupefaction, hysteria and insanity, and possession – whether divine or demonic (Dodds, 1965, p. 70–72). The Septuagint renders the deep sleep (*tardema*) of Abraham (Gen. 15.12) and Daniel's trembling (Dan. 10: 7) an *ekstasis*. In fact, the word *ekstasis* occurs twenty-seven times in the Septuagint to translate eleven different Hebrew words. It is only with Plotinus that it comes to signify mystical union and probably entered the Christian lexicon with Tertullian, who uses it in his *Adversus Marcionum* (VI. 22. 5).[42] He defines it, in relation to dreams, as an *amentia*, a flight of the mind (*De Anima* MPL II: 725b) (cited in Gilson, 1940, p. 215, n. 6; cf. De Brabander, 2012). With Bernard of Clairvaux and the early Cistercians, this flight becomes an *excessus* which signifies, in a general way, exceeding limits, specifically in order to attain the mystical state.[43] This includes taking a person beyond thought itself (*abductio interioris sensus*) (Gilson, 1940, p. 237, n. 156). With William of St Thierry, the experience of the mystical is understood as something that develops gradually and is intrinsically a part of faith (Brooke, 1964). Recently, Cristiana Cimino has suggested that "the theme of 'ecstatic' opening pervades the entire 20th century" (Cimino, 2017, p. 17).

For Heidegger, the primordial ecstasy or "out-of-oneself" is temporality (*Zeitlichkeit*).

> The future, the character of having been, and the Present, show the phenomenal characteristics of the "towards-oneself," the "back-to," and the "letting-oneself-be-encountered-*by*." The phenomena of the "towards . . . ," and "to . . . ," and the "alongside . . . ," make temporality manifest as the ἐκστατικόν pure and simple. *Temporality is the primordial "outside-of-itself" in and for itself.* We therefore call the phenomenon of the future, the character of having been, and the Present, the "ecstasies" of temporality.[44]
>
> SZ 328–9

Heidegger says that ecstasy allows time to emerge (*entspringen*) or unfold in an interwoven threefold structure of past, present, and future (SZ 329). While dwelling in time is the fundamental way in which Dasein transcends itself, by choosing the Greek word *ekstasis* to describe originary time, as opposed to sequential time (our everyday way of thinking about time), Heidegger is suggesting that displacement or "stepping beyond itself" is a key function of being, the meaning of the ground of Dasein. In other words, to say we exist "ecstatically" is to refer to the way in which being opens and transcends itself (SZ 338). In fact, the word existence itself comes, via the Latin *existere* (to appear; to become), from *ex-stare* (to stand out). That is to say, its etymology exactly parallels the Greek *ekstatikon* (*ek-stasis*). Yet this fundamental aspect of existence as transcending is normally overlooked.

This view may, at first, seem antithetical to that of Aristotle, as in keeping with medical writers, he habitually uses the word *ekstasis* to mean what Plato would consider human madness. However, Aristotle also makes clear the link between the ecstatic as displacement, and time (Arist. Phys. 22b.15, quoted in Krell, 2016).

According to Fann (2016), in the *Phaedrus*, philosophy itself is presented as a kind of madness.[45] That is to say, it is not just that philosophy may sometimes be considered madness by people that do not understand it, but that the philosophical soul is not entirely in rational control of philosophical thought but in a state of mind that can fairly be defined as madness – and that the philosophical life is arranged in order to visit or revisit this state of mind. In other words, madness is at the center of the best human life; namely, the philosophical life. The madness of philosophical thought involves not knowing what to do (*aporein*) (Arist.

Top. 145b 16). It is a kind of puzzle which the philosopher is trying to solve (Arist. N.E. 1145b 2). But *aporia* also means the absence of a way through as, for example, in the case of rugged terrain. This idea of not knowing what to do or coming to a dead end, is reflected in Heidegger's work as a whole which, in Schürmann's words, is "unified solely by a path in thinking, a path that, in a sense, leads nowhere" (Schürmann, 2008, p. 63). In the epigraph to Heidegger's *Holzwege* (woodpaths), the title he gave to the fifth volume of his collected works,[46] we read:

> In the wood are paths which mostly wind along until they end quite suddenly in an impenetrable thicket. They are called "woodpaths." Each goes its peculiar way, but in the same forest. Often it seems as though one were like another. Yet it only seems so. Wood cutters and forest rangers are familiar with these paths. They know what it means to be on a woodpath.
>
> (Heidegger, 1950, p. 1, quoted by Schürmann, 2008, p. 63)

Hannah Arendt considered that the metaphor of woodpaths hit upon something essential in Heidegger's philosophy. What Schürmann added to this was the idea that this was true not only in relation to Heidegger's itinerary of thinking but also in terms of the itinerary of being.[47]

> The "itinerary of Being" – Heidegger is particularly fond of phrases like this, but they are not without traps – would itself be something like a woodpath . . .
>
> That the itinerary of the question of Being resembles woodpaths also means that the entire path of philosophy since the Greeks is in errancy – not an error, but a wandering. This, too, has tremendous consequences, which I only gesture toward here: "Who thinks greatly must err greatly" (Heidegger *Aus der Erfahrung des Denkens*, GA 13, p. 81).
>
> Schürmann, 2008, pp. 63–64.

Woodcutters do not intentionally make paths in the forest. They come about merely as a result of felling trees. The clearings they open up are not designed to lead anywhere, though some may. But others lead to a dead end. Heidegger is suggesting that thinking philosophically opens up tracks in which one might get a hint or indication of that mystery which permeates the everyday world, but generally goes unnoticed because of its "simplicity and familiarity" (P.I. 129).[48] And that the reason for being on the "path of thinking" is not to arrive at a specific destination, because the direction thought takes is always unknown. Thinking about being does not have a *telos* in mind and does not proceed logically. It is a kind of wandering, meandering form of thinking, not dependent solely on what is conscious. Yet here, as it were, one might stumble across a clearing in which we are able to catch a glimpse of things in the light of our understanding of being (*die Lichtung des Seins*).

Conclusion

The question of madness is always a question about exceedance, and thus of limits. This not only connects it to Oedipus, a point that Lacan brought into full view (*forclusion*), but also ties it to the question of the mystical (de Certeau, 2013). In so doing, something of the mystery and transcendence of being is revealed. This is seen in the way the rules of language are transgressed in an attempt to grasp the ungraspable.[49] Indeed, mystical texts are often inscrutable, at times aphoristic, frequently indirect, deeply ambiguous and obscure, recurrently inaccessible and unfinished (cf. Lévy-Valensi, 1956). These literary characteristics are part of a peculiar way of speaking in which "knowing" is gradually eclipsed. The disappearance of meaning that penetrates these texts, nevertheless, has its own peculiar logic, which points beyond itself thus opening up a new perspective "at the limit of the world" (T 5.632).

For Plato, prophecy and participation in the mysteries disclose this "beyond," as both overstep the limit of rationality (*logos*). In ambiguous, enigmatic utterances, the prophets were thought to speak a truth that was not fully accessible but was, nonetheless, able to be interpreted and made relevant to everyday events within a specific community. The Oracle spoke, that is to say, a "word" for the here and now. Likewise, the catharsis which resulted from the trances induced during the sacred rites (the mysteries) was probably not unconnected to the temporary liberation from social difference that the devotee experienced. That is to say, it had an impact (a blessing) in terms of everyday life. The development of an inspirational theory of poetry, which begins mildly and is only later seen as a frenzied state, is first mentioned by Democritus in fr. 17,18 (Dodds, 1959, p. 101 n.125) and may well itself have been influenced by the Dionysian rites. The Muses were thought to endow the poet with a knowledge of the truth, which likened him to the prophet (Vicaire, 1963). Yet even here, the true value and "blessing" of poetry, in antiquity, lay in its ethical dimension (*paideia*).

The passion of good *erōs* mirrors the kind of thinking that is central to philosophy. Of course, philosophy – as its conventional etymology would suggest – is a kind of love (*philia*). But it is also a form of madness, because it necessarily leads us to 'step beyond' (*ek-stasis*) rationality (Schürmann, 2008, p. 83). But it is a 'sane madness' and a 'wise foolishness' (St Paul), as the uncharted course that it follows, allows something other than conscious thought to show itself. Moreover, if Heidegger's development of Aristotle is legitimate, time – which is constitutive of being – is not really sequential but a simultaneous movement from the past to the present to the future. The present moment, from inside of which we view our existence, is fundamentally ecstatic.[50]

More often than not, those possessed of madness are written off by the wise and learned. Their utterances, as those of the poet and the seer, in antiquity, seem obscure; their behavior, like that of the ascetic, frequently strange and challenging. "Touched," absurd and out of place, they may be ridiculed and derided, as indeed was Socrates, as well as many of the Old Testament prophets, and the "fools for Christ." Yet might not these "outsiders," in their fragility, open up to us manifold new paths of thinking, new horizons, and something of the unbounded-ness of language? And in so doing, might they not clear a space for a glimpse of the "truth of unreason," to use Foucault's idiom, to emerge; and for being itself, in its primordial transcending, to be disclosed in the mystery of the everyday? For "to be" means, pre-eminently, to be "out-of-it."

Abbreviations

Plat. Apol.	Plato. *Apology* in Plato. *Euthyphro. Apology. Crito. Phaedo. Phaedrus* (trans.) H. North Fowler. Loeb Classical Library 36. Cambridge, MA: Harvard University Press, 1914.
Plat. Crat.	Plato. Cratylus in *Plato. Cratylus. Parmenides. Greater Hippias. Lesser Hippias* (trans.) H. N. Fowler. Loeb Classical Library 167. Cambridge, MA: Harvard University Press, 1926.
Plat. Ion	Plato. Ion in *Plato. Statesman. Philebus. Ion* (trans.) Harold North Fowler, W. R. M. Lamb. Loeb Classical Library 164. Cambridge, MA: Harvard University Press, 1925.
Plat. Phaed.	Plato. *Phaedrus* op.cit.
Plat. Phileb.	Plato. *Philebus* op.cit.
Plat. Sym.	Plato. *Symposium* in *Plato. Lysis. Symposium. Gorgias* (trans.) W. R. M. Lamb. Loeb Classical Library 166. Cambridge, MA: Harvard University Press, 1925.
Plat. Theaet.	Plato. Theaetetus in *Plato. Theaetetus. Sophist* (trans.) H.N. Fowler. Loeb Classical Library 123. Cambridge, MA: Harvard University Press, 1921.
Plat. Theag.	Plato. Theages in *Plato. Charmides. Alcibiades I and II. Hipparchus. The Lovers. Theages. Minos. Epinomis* (trans.) W. R. M. Lamb. Loeb Classical Library 201. Cambridge, MA: Harvard University Press, 1927.
Plat. Tim.	Plato. Timaeus in *Plato. Timaeus. Critias. Cleitophon. Menexenus. Epistles* (trans.) R. G. Bury. Loeb Classical Library 234. Cambridge, MA: Harvard University Press, 1929.
Arist. Met.	Aristotle. Metaphysics in *Aristotle. Metaphysics, Volume II: Books 10–14. Oeconomica. Magna Moralia* (trans.) H. Tredennick, G. Cyril Armstrong. Loeb Classical Library 287. Cambridge, MA: Harvard University Press, 1935.
Arist. Nic. Eth.	Aristotle. *Nicomachean Ethics* (trans.) H. Rackham. Loeb Classical Library 73. Cambridge, MA: Harvard University Press, 1926.
Arist. Phys.	Aristotle. Physics in *Aristotle. Physics*, Volume I: Books 1–4 (trans.) P. H. Wicksteed and F. M. Cornford. Loeb Classical Library 228. Cambridge, MA: Harvard University Press, 1957.

Arist. Top.   Aristotle. *Topica* in *Posterior Analytics. Topica.* (trans.) H. Tredennick and E. S. Forster. Loeb Classical Library 391. Cambridge, MA: Harvard University Press, 1960.

Apoph. Pat.   Apophthegmata Patrum. J.P. Migne (Ed.) *Patrologiae Cursus Completus, Series Graeca* LXV. 121 (Eng.) The Sayings of the Desert Fathers. The Alphabetical Collection (trans.) B. Ward. London and Oxford: Mowbray, 1981.

Cic. Pro Archia   Cicero. Pro Archia in *Cicero. Pro Archia. Post Reditum in Senatu. Post Reditum ad Quirites. De Domo Sua. De Haruspicum Responsis. Pro Plancio* (trans.) N. H. Watts. Loeb Classical Library 158. Cambridge, MA: Harvard University Press, 1923.

Xen. Mem.   Xenophon. Memorabilia in *Xenophon. Memorabilia. Oeconomicus. Symposium. Apology* (trans.) E. C. Marchant and O. J. Todd, revised by J. Henderson. Loeb Classical Library 168. Cambridge, MA: Harvard University Press, 2013.

DL   Diogenes Laertius. *Lives of Eminent Philosophers*. Vol II. (trans.) R.D. Hicks. Loeb Classical Library 185. London: William Heinemann Ltd and Cambridge MA: Harvard University Press, 1950.

Contra Cels.   Origen. *Contra Celsum*. Sources Chrétiennes 132. Paris: Cerf, 1967.

Basil Ep.   *St. Basil. Letters, I*: Letters 1–58 (trans.) R. J. Deferrari. Loeb Classical Library 190. Cambridge, MA: Harvard University Press, 1926.

Clim. scal.   Joannes Climacus. *Scala paradisi*. Migne Patrologiae Graecae 88, 632–1208. (Eng.). John Climacus. *The Ladder of Divine Ascent* (trans.) C. Luibheid and N. Russell. London: SPCK, 1982.

Pall. h. Laus.   Palladius. *Lausiac History* in *La Storia Lausica* (ed.) G.J.M. Bartelink. Milan: Fondazione Lorenzo Valla. Arnoldo Mondadori Editore.

Pleroph.   John Rufus. Plerophories. *Jean Rufus. Plérophories* (ed.) F. Nau. Patrologia Orientalis VIII (1). No 36. Turnhout: Brepols.

Rel. Hist.   Theodoret. Religious History. Théodort de Cyr. Histoire des Moines de Syrie. 2 vols, (eds.) P. Canivet and A. Leroy-Molinghen. Sources Chrétiennes No 234 and 257. Paris: Les Éditions du Cerf, 1977, 1979.

V   Thomas Aquinas. *Quaestiones Disputate de Veritate* (ed.) R.M. Spiazzi. Rome: Marietti, 1949.

ST   Thomas Aquinas, *Summa Theologiae*. Vol. 1. London: Eyre & Spottiswoode, 1963.

DN   Pseudo Dionysius. *The Divine Names in Pseudo Dionysius. The Complete Works* 47–132 (trans.) C. Luibheid. New York: Paulist Press, 1987.

Freud SE II   Breuer, J. and Freud, S. (1893–1985). *Studies in Hysteria. The Standard Editor of the Complete Psychological Works of Sigmund Freud* II (trans. and ed.) J. Strachey. London: The Hogarth press and Institute of Psycho-Analysis.

Freud SE VII   Freud, S. (1920). Three Essays on the Theory of Sexuality *The Standard Editor of the Complete Psychological Works of Sigmund Freud* VII, pp. 125–172 (trans. and ed.) J. Strachey. London: The Hogarth press and Institute of Psycho-Analysis.

Freud SE XII   Freud, S. (1914). Remembering, Repeating and Working-Through (Further Recommendations on the Technique of Psycho-Analysis II) *The Standard Editor of the Complete Psychological Works of Sigmund Freud* XII, 145–156 (trans. and ed.) J. Strachey. London: The Hogarth press and Institute of Psycho-Analysis.

Freud SE XIII   Freud, S. (1912–13). *Totem and Taboo. The Standard Editor of the Complete Psychological Works of Sigmund Freud* XIII (trans. and ed.) J. Strachey. London: The Hogarth press and Institute of Psycho-Analysis.

Freud SE XIV   Freud, S. (1919 [1915]). Mourning and Melancholia (1917 [1915]) *The Standard Edition of the Complete Psychological Works of Sigmund Freud* XIV, 237–258 (trans. and ed.) J. Strachey. London: The Hogarth press and Institute of Psycho-Analysis.

Freud SE XVIII   Freud, S. (1921). Group Psychology and the Analysis of the Ego. The Standard Editor of the Complete Psychological Works of Sigmund Freud XVIII, 69–133 (trans. and ed.) J. Strachey. London: The Hogarth Press and Institute of Psycho-Analysis.

Freud SE XX   Freud, S. (1924). An Autobiographical Study *The Standard Editor of the Complete Psychological Works of Sigmund Freud* XX, 7–76 (trans. and ed.) J. Strachey. London: The Hogarth press and Institute of Psycho-Analysis.

Freud SE XXIII   Freud, S. (1938). An Outline of Psycho-Analysis *The Standard Edition of the Complete Psychological Works of Sigmund Freud* Vol XXIII, 144–207 (trans. and ed.) J. Strachey. London: Hogarth Press and the Institute of Psycho-Analysis.

GA   Heidegger, M. *Aus der Erfahrung des Denkens (1910–1976).* Gesamtausgabe 13. Verlag Vittorio Klostermann, 1983.

SZ   Heidegger, M. (1990). *Being and Time* (trans.) J. Macquarrie and E. Robinson. Oxford: Basil Blackwell.

PI   Wittgenstein, L. *Philosophical Investigations* (trans.) G.E.M. Anscombe. Oxford: Blackwell, 1999.

T   Wittgenstein, L. *Tractatus Logico-Philosophicus* (trans.) D.F. Pears and B.F. McGuinness. London: Routledge, 1988.

Notes

1 The expression is that of the classical scholar Werner Jaeger (1943, p. 343) who formed this opinion based on an analysis of the *Republic* 571–572. Here "the divine Plato," to use Freud's expression, describes the way incestuous desires surface in dreams. Given that Freud constructed psychoanalysis in relation to Greek myth (Oedipus) and that, more than any other philosopher – including Aristotle, Augustine, Descartes and Immanuel Kant – Plato played a vital role in his work, it may be worth considering seriously his view of divine madness and its gifts (Rottenberg, 2019).

2 Although Lacan restricts the word "mad" to psychosis (Lacan, 1993), he nonetheless does not see madness (*folie*) as entirely negative. In fact, he praises Henri Ey for preserving the term (Lacan, 2006; cf. Vanheule, 2017).

3 ὅτι δὲ ἀτοπώτατός εἰμι καὶ ποιῶ τοὺς ἀνθρώπους ἀπορεῖν.

4 *Mōros* can mean dull or sluggish and in relation to the mind, stupid, silly, foolish; *mōria*, folly.

5 For the verb *mōrainō* (Matt. 5.13/Lk. 14.34); for the condemnation of *mōre* (Matt. 5.22); for the evaluation of the builders and virgins in the parables (Matt. 7.24–27; 25.1–13); for the description of the Pharisees as *mōroi kai tuphloi* (fools and blind) (Matt. 23.17).

6 Cynicism seems to have started in the second half of the 4th century B.C. and continued to develop, through a number of different phases, to the end of the Roman empire. Dudley (1937) shows its breadth and complexity and makes it clear that it would be a mistake to imagine it was limited to the vagrant ascetic form associated with Diogenes.

7 This sets Cynicism firmly within the famous Socratic dictum "know thyself." As Pierre Hadot puts it: "*Se connaître comme non-sage (c'est-à-dire non comme sophos, mais comme philo-sophos, comme en marche vers la sagesse), ou bien se connaître en son être essential (c'est-à-dire séparer ce qui n'est pas nous de ce qui est nons-mêmes), ou bien se connaître en son veritable état moral (c'est-à-dire examiner sa conscience)*" (Hadot, 1987, p. 31; on the background to the term "know thyself," see Courcelle, 1975). The refusal by the philosopher to identify himself as a sage also has some resonance with Lacan's notion that imaginary self-knowledge must be challenged, as it is fundamentally a misrecognition based on the ego (Lacan, 2006).

8 In fact, an apophatic note can be detected throughout the *Tractatus*. There we read, for example, "My propositions serve as elucidations in the following way: anyone who understands me eventually recognizes them as nonsensical, when he has used them – as steps – to climb up beyond them. (He must, so to speak, throw away the ladder after he has climbed up it.) He must transcend these propositions, and then he will see the world aright. What we cannot speak about we must pass over in silence" (T. 6. 54–7).

9 Caputo noticed how close Heidegger's view of the nothing (*das Nichts*) was to that expressed by Meister Eckhart's in his treatise *Von Abgeschiedenheit* (on detachment). Cf. Caputo (1986, pp. 10–11, 271, n. 4).

10 The very notion of mystical discourse brings to the fore the question of how we might speak about that which lies beyond the bounded whole (Wittgenstein) and cannot be symbolised (Lacan). As pseudo Denys puts it: "This is why we must not dare to resort to words or conceptions concerning that hidden divinity which transcends being . . . Since the unknowing of what is beyond being is something above and beyond speech, mind, or being itself, one should ascribe to it an understanding beyond being"; and "if all knowledge is of that which is and is limited to the realm of the existent, then whatever transcends being must also transcend knowledge" (DN 588A; 593A).

11 Both in its provenance and in its meaning, the expression, which appears in a wide variety of versions, is fraught with difficulty. It is even uncertain whether it originates with Socrates. For a fascinating and erudite review of the matter, see Fine (2008).

12 Dibelius (1937) suggested a Cynic background to I Thess. II. More recently, Bornkamm lent his support to this idea (cited in Malherbe, 1970).

13 Theodoret (Rel. Hist.) gives examples of a number of Syrian monks dressing in rags or skins, living in the open air or in caves or holes in the ground, wearing chains, and sleeping on the ground. They could be threatening and even dangerous in their criticism of the intuitional Church (Urbainczyk, 2002).

14 Bousset did the pioneering work in analyzing the Apophthegmata in its various collections, though not the Arabic version. Further work was done by Guy (1962). As a genre, these sayings may have a direct link to the *chreiae* associated with Diogenes and the other Cynic philosophers.

15 The notion of interior or psychic "work" was one of the many fundamentally religious ideas taken up by Freud. This family resemblance, to use Wittgenstein's phrase (Wittgenstein P.I. 65–71), between the "work of the soul" and psychoanalysis can be seen clearly not only in the way Freud referred to unconscious "working through" (*Durcharbeitung* or *Durcharbeiten*; cf. SE II, pp. 288, 291; SE XII, p. 155; SE XX, p. 159) and the "work of mourning" (*Trauerarbeit*; cf. SE II, p. 162; SE XIV, pp. 245, 255), but more fundamentally in his choice of the word *Psychoanalyse* itself. *Psuchē* is usually translated as soul (*anima* in Latin) to distinguish it not only from the body (*soma*) – or when described in a pejorative sense, from the flesh (*sarx*) – but also from *nous* (Latin *mens*, intellect). Freud seems to have been aware of this ambiguity and grappled with it in his discussion of the equivalence of the German *Geist* (spirit) and *Seele* (soul), terms he uses almost interchangeably (cf. Strachey's note in SE XXIII, p. 114).

16 A number of the Church Fathers, including Clement of Alexandria, Origen, and Gregory of Nyssa, contrast the drunkenness of madness caused by drinking wine with the *nēphalios methē* (sober drunkenness) or "sane madness" of mystical union. This was discussed in a monograph by Hans Lewy (1929).

17 The Latin is rendered in Migne's edition as "*stultum simulabat . . . fatuis est . . . fatuitatem acquirerem.*"

18 For an unusual reading of this text, see de Certeau, 1982, p. 48ff).

19 Špidlík's (1963) derivation of *salos* from the Syriac was repeated by Bartelink in 1974, but Guillaumont was not convinced. More recently, Ivanov (2006; originally published in Russian in 1994) has reviewed the literature and others, notably Krueger (1996), largely repeat his conclusions.

20 Nau translates it as *l'idiot* (n. 1, p. 178).

21 We find this apophatic view of knowledge and not knowing, which we have already noted in the Cynics and in Plato's Socrates, significantly developed in a number of monastic writers in late antiquity, notably in Evagrius Ponticus. What is described here as a descent into the unlimited or infinite ignorance is, according to Wensinck, synonymous with the unconscious. For differing readings of this concept and particularly in its relationship to *apophasis*, see Guillaumont (1985), Wensinck (1923), and Hausherr (1959, 1960).

22 There were, of course, cases of genuine insanity among the early monks, including sexual obsessions and 'pathological cases of hatred' (Clim. scal. 8, cited in Brown 1988, p. 230), symptoms of which were often accompanied by hallucination (Canivet, 1962).

23 Krueger (1996) gives some examples in which *salos* is used to describe genuine as opposed to simulated madness. But it seems to me that he does this principally in order to build his argument that the fool cannot be thought a distinct category of asceticism. However, when the wider context of mad behaviour is taken into account, particularly in the context of Cynicism, his argument here seems rather weak.

24 *Apatheia* plays an important role in ethics from the Cynics on. It is particularly developed by Stoic writers, and then taken up again in Neoplatonic thought, in Evagrius and Dorotheos of Gaza.

25 The Roman physician, Caelius Aurelianus, refers to this dual idea of madness (*duplicem furorem*), set out by Plato in the *Phaedrus*: *Unum fieri mentis intentione ex corporis causa vel origine, alterum divinum sive immissum* (Drabkin, 1950, p. 265).

26 Indirectly, the cult of Dionysus is linked to that of Asklepios, in which cures were sought through the ritual of incubation (Wickkister, 2008). It was a practice that continued in Christianity. For cures by Christian martyrs according to the Coptic passions, see Banmeister (1972). Later, we find Bernard of Clairvaux describing mystical ecstasy as a kind of sleep (*dormitio, somnus, sopor*) (Gilson, 1940).

27 For the figure of Socrates as the lover (*erotikos*), see also Xen. Mem. 11, 6, 28.

28 For Plato, the soul (*psuchē*) is divided into three parts. He calls these the rational (*logistikon*), the spirited (*thumoeidēs*) and the appetitive (*epithumētikon*) (Rep. ix, 580d–581a; Phaed. 246a–b, 253c–255b; and Tim. 9d–72d).

29 Freud, in the preface to the 1920 edition of the *Three Essays on the Theory of Sexuality* wrote that he considered Plato's *erōs* a notion identical to the libido of psychoanalysis ('*Sexualität der Psychoanalyse mit dem Eros des göttlichen Plato zusammentriff'* Freud SE VII, p. 134). He repeated this again in 1921 (SE XVIII: 91) and in 1924 (SE XX: 24). He relied heavily, for this position, on a grossly inaccurate paper by Nachmansohn (1915), which he cited, and to a lesser extent on one by Pfister (1921) which was largely derivative of it. Nachmansohn's description of Plato's doctrine was based almost exclusively on a discussion of the *Symposium*, and his conclusions are not supported by a scholarly reading of Plato's work (Stok, 2007). Specifically, he made no mention of the distinction between *erōs* and *philia*. As Santas notes, "Freud did himself no favour relying on these papers" (Santas, 1988, p. 155).

30 In a fascinating paper, Boysen (2018) reads Plato's position both as a development in his philosophy and as parallel to the notion of the *pharmakon* as both poison and medicine (cf. Derrida, 1968).

31 See e.g. Crat. 396–397; and Phaed. 265.

32 For the literary background, see Sikes (1931), Tigerstedt (1970) and Vicaire (1963).

33 "And yet we have it on the highest and most learned authority that while other arts are matters of science and formula and technique, poetry depends solely upon an inborn faculty, is evoked by a purely mental activity, and is infused with a strange supernatural inspiration (*quasi divino quodam spiritu inflari*). Rightly, then, did our great Ennius call poets 'holy' (*sanctos*), for they seem recommended to us by the benign bestowal of God" (Cic. Pro Archia VIII. 18).

34 Although it is not easy historically to draw a sharp line between Christian and Platonic mysticism (Festugière, 1954) or eroticism (Armstrong, 1961), Origen and Gregory of Nyssa seem to have been the first Christian authors to adopt erotic imagery to describe the mystical life. But in keeping with biblical symbolism, this is set firmly within the context of the relationship between the community (Israel; the Church) – rather than the individual soul – and the divine (Crouzel, 1961). This social, ecclesial dimension re-appears in Bernard's sermons on the Canticle.

35 Lacan, however, would not see this as madness. In fact, he thought Schreber's text totally lacked the quality he admired in John of the Cross.

36 Hölderlin did, in fact, suffer from bouts of madness (Hamburger, 2004). Rilke, much of whose poetry has a mystical dimension, had a relationship with Lou Andreas-Salomé from whom he gained a knowledge of psychoanalysis.

37 See Laplanche (1961). This idea is mirrored in Foucault's notion that it is the artist's excess in which the work of art is engulfed.

38 The fragments are published in Diels (1906) I, pp. 113–126, and Coxon (1986) gives the text with translation and commentary.

39 The key texts in Thomas are *V* I, 1–2 and *ST* I, q. 16. Nathan Strunk (n.d.) reviews this passage in Heidegger very usefully, citing Aertsen (1991): *transcendens* suggests a kind of surpassing. "What is transcended are the special modes of being that Aristotle called the 'categories,' in the sense that the transcendentals are not restricted to one determinate category. 'Being' and its 'concomitant conditions,' such as 'one,' 'true' and 'good,' 'go through (*circumeunt*) all the categories' (to use an expression of Thomas Aquinas)" (Aertsen, 1991, p. 130).

40 Plato makes explicit references to Corybantic rites in six of his dialogues. Wasmuth (2015) notices that in all but one an analogy is drawn between these rites and some kind of logos. Plato's use of Corybantic analogies is thus quite extensive. Indeed, according to Linforth (1946a), Plato is our "principal witness concerning Corybantic rites and their function." Ecstatic features, including frenzied dancing, also characterised some of the early Old Testament prophets who gave the impression of being mad. But gradually, ecstasy gave way to a focus on the word e.g. 1 Sam. 10.10f, 19.23f.

41 On *ekstasis*, see p. 7, 58, 68, 75, 119f, 160f, and 203.

42 *In spiritu enim homo constitutus, praesertim cum gloriam dei conspicit, vel cum per ipsum deus loquitur, necesse est excidat sensu, obumbratus scilicet virtute divina, de quo inter nos et psychicos quaestio est.*

43 Gilson points out that Bernard rarely uses the word *extasis*. "He uses it, however, to designate the state in which the corporeal senses cease to exercise their functions. In this sense it belongs to the genus *excessus*" (Gilson, 1940, p. 237, n. 156).

44 "*Zukunft, Gewesenheit, Gegenwart zeigen die phänomenalen Charaktere des 'Auf-sich-zu,' des 'Zurück auf,' des 'Begegnenlassens von.' Die Phänomene des zu . . . , auf . . . , bei . . . , offenbaren die Zeitlichkeit als das ἐκστατικόν schlechthin. Zeitlichkeit ist das ursprüngliche 'Außer-sich' an und für sich selbst. Wir nennen daher die charakterisierten Phänomene Zukunft, Gewesenheit, Gegenwart die Ekstasen der Zeitlichkeit. Sie ist nicht vordem ein Seiendes, das erst aus sich heraustritt, sondern ihr Wesen ist Zeitigung in der Einheit der Ekstasen.*"

45 The meaning of the Greek word *philosophia*, and its kindred terms, is remarkably elastic. We can see, from its first known use in fragment 35 of Heraclitus (Diels, 1906) right through to John Chrysostom, that neither of its component parts remained static for very long (Malingrey, 1961).

46 This volume contains his published works from 1910–1976.

47 While Arendt considered that while the metaphor of the woodpath indicated something essential in Heidegger's thought, it was not because the paths of thought came to dead ends. "Not, as one may at first think, that someone had gotten into a dead-end trail, but rather that someone, like the woodcutter whose occupation lies in the woods, treads paths that he has himself beaten; and clearing the path belongs no less to his line of work than felling trees" (Arendt, 1971, p. 51).

48 "The aspects of things which are most important for us are hidden because of their simplicity and familiarity. (One is unable to notice something – because it is always before one's eyes.)" (P.I. 129).

49 For Heidegger, language is most eminently itself in poetry because in poetry, language speaks for itself. The poet is only the transmitter of language (D'hert, 1974).

50 Heidegger calls the present the moment of vision (*Er meint die entschlossene, aber in der Erschlossenheit gehaltene Entrückung des Daseins an das, was in der Situation an besorgbaren Möglichkeiten, Umständen begegnet* SZ 338). See Macquarrie's note 3 (SZ: 338) on *entrücken* ("to move away," "to carry away," or figuratively, "to be carried away" as in rapture).

References

Aertsen, J. (1991). The medieval doctrine of the transcendentals: The current state of research. *Bulletin de philosophie médiévale, 33*, 130–147.

Arendt, H. (1971, October 21). Martin Heidegger at eighty. *The New York Review of Books.*

Armstrong, A. H. (1961). Platonic Eros and Christian Agape. *The Downside Review, 79*, 105–121.

Attridge, H. W. (1976). *First-century cynicism in the epistles of Heraclitus. Harvard theological studies XXIX.* Missoula, MT: Scholars Press for the Harvard Theological Review.

Banmeister, T. (1972). *Martyr invictus. Der Martyrer als Sinnbild der Erlösung in der Legende und im Kult der frühen koptischen Kirche. Zur Kontinuität des ägyptischen Denkens Forschungen zur Volkskunde* (Vol. 46). Münster: Regensberg.

Billault, A. (2002). La folie poétique: remarques sur les conceptions grecques de l'inspiration. *Bulletin de l'Association Guillaume Budé: Lettres d'humanité, 61*, 18–35.

Bousset, W. (1923). *Apophthegmata. Textüberlieferung und Charakter der Apophthegmata Patrum. Zur Überlieferung der Vita Pachomii Euagriou-Studien.* Tübingen: Verlag von J. C. B. Mohr (Paul Siebeck).

Boysen, B. (2018). Poetry, philosophy, and madness in Plato. *Res Cogitans, 13*(1), 154–184.

Brooke, O. (1964). Faith and mystical experience in William of St Thierry. *The Downside Review, 82*, 93–102.

Brown, P. (1988). *Society and the holy in late antiquity.* London: Faber and Faber.

Campbell, R. (Trans.). (1972). *The poems of St John of the cross. The Spanish text with a translation.* London: Harvill Press.

Canivet, P. (1962). Erreurs de spiritualité et troubles psychiques. À propos d'un passage de la Vie de s. Théodose par Théodore de Pétra (530). *Recherches de science religieuse, 50*, 161–205.

Caputo, J. D. (1986). *The mystical element in Heidegger's thought.* New York: Fordham University Press.

Cimino, C. (2017). The Ek-static love. A feminine ethical perspective. *Vestigia, 1*, 10–19. http://inppjournal.org.uk/vestigia-11/.

Courcelle, P. (1975). *Connais-toi toi-même. De Socrate à saint Bernard.* Paris: Études Augustiniennes.

Coxon, A. H. (Ed. & Trans.). (1986). *The fragments of Parmenides. A critical text with introduction, translation, the ancient testimonia and a commentary.* Assen & Maastricht: Van Gorcum.

Crouzel, H. (1961). *Origène et la "Connaissance Mystique".* Paris: Desclée de Brouwer.

De Brabander, K. (2012). Tertullian's theory of dreams (De Anima 45–49). Some observations towards a better understanding. In B. J. Koet (Ed.), *Dreams as divine communication in Christianity. From Hermas to Aquinas.* Leuven: Peeters Publishers.

de Certeau, M. (1982). *La Fable mystique.* Paris: Gallimard.

de Certeau, M. (2013). *La Fable mystique XVIᵉ – XVIIᵉ II.* Paris: Gallimard.

Delatte, A. (1934). Les conceptions de l'enthousiasme chez les philosophes présocratiques. *L'Antiquité Classique, 3*(1), 5–79.

Derrida, J. (1968). La pharmacie de Platon. *Tel Quel, 32*, 3–48, 33, 18–59.

D'hert, I. (1974). *Wittgenstein's relevance for theology.* Bern: Peter Lang.

Dibelius, M. (1937). An die Thessalonicher I. II. An die Philipper. *Handbuch zum Neuen Testament, 11*, 7–11. Tubingen: Mohr.

Diels, H. (1906). *Die Fragmente der Vorsokratiker I*. Berlin: Weidmannsche Buchhandlung.

Dodds, E. R. (1959). *The Greeks and the irrational*. Berkeley and Los Angeles: University of California Press.

Dodds, E. R. (1965). *Pagan and Christian in an age of anxiety*. Cambridge: Cambridge University Press.

Drabkin, I. E. (Ed. & Trans.). (1950). *Caelius Aurelianus: On acute diseases and on chronic diseases*. Chicago, IL: University of Chicago Press.

Dudley, D. (1937). *A history of cynicism. From Diogenes to the 6th century A.D.* London: Methuen & Co. Ltd.

Fann, L. (2016). *Love and madness in Plato's Phaedrus*. A Thesis Submitted for the Degree of PhD at the University of St Andrews. http://hdl.handle.net/10023/8424.

Fascher, E. (1927). *PROPHĒTĒS: Eine sprach und religion geschichliche Unterspuchung*. Geissen: Alfred Töpelmann.

Festugière, A.-J. (1954). *Personal religion among the Greeks*. Berkeley & Los Angeles: University of California Press.

Festugière, A.-J. (Ed.). (1974). *Vie de Syméon le Fou et Vie de Jean de Chypre*. Paris: P. Geuthner.

Fine, G. (2008). Does Socrates claim to know the he knows nothing? In B. Inwood (Ed.), *Oxford studies in ancient philosophy* (Vol. XXXV, pp. 49–88). Oxford: Oxford University Press.

Foucault, M. (2014). *On the government of the living. Lectures at the Collège de France 1979–1980* (G. Burchell, Trans.). Basingstoke: Palgrave Macmillan.

Gadamer, H.-G. (1997). *Gadamer on Celan. "Who Am I and Who Are You?" and other essays* (R. Heinemann & B. Krajewski, Trans. & Eds.), New York: State University of New York Press.

Gibb, H. O. (1941). *"Torheit" und "Rätsel" im Neuen Testament: Der antinomische Strukturcharakter der neutestamentlichen Botschaft*. Stuttgart: Kohlhammer.

Gilson, E. (1940). *The mystical theology of Saint Bernard* (A.H.C. Downes, Trans.). London: Sheed & Ward.

Goulet-Cazé, M.-O. (1986). *L'Ascèse Cynique. Un commentaire de Diogène Laërce VI 70–71*. Paris: J. Vrin.

Guillaumont, A. (1985). Les Six Centuries des "Kephalaia Gnostica" d'Évagre Le Pontique. *Patrologia Orientalis, Tome XXVIII*(134). Turnhout: Editions Brepols.

Guillaumont, A. (1996). La Folie Simuée, une Forme d'Anachorèse. In *Études sur la Spiritualité de l'Orient Chrétien* (pp. 125–150). Bégrolles-en-Mauges: Annaye de Bellefontaine.

Guy, J.-C. (1962). *Recherches sur la tradition Grecque des Apophthegmata Patrum*. Bruxelles: Société des Bollandistes.

Hadot, P. (1987). *Exercices Spirituels et Philosophie Antique*. Paris: Études Augustiniennes.

Hamburger, M. (2004). Introduction. In *Friedrich Hölderlin. Poems and fragments* (M. Hamburger, Trans., pp. 23–54). London: Anvil Press Poetry.

Hausherr, I. (1959). Ignorance infini. *Orientalia Christiana Periodica, XXV*, 44–52.

Hausherr, I. (1960). *Les Leçons d'un Contemplatif. Le Traité de l'Oraison d'Evagre le Pontique*. Paris: Beauchesne et ses fils.

Heidegger, M. (1950). *Holzwege*. Frankfurt am Main: Vittorio Klostermann.

Heidegger, M. (1959). *An introduction to metaphysics*. New Haven: Yale University Press.

Ivanov, S. A. (2006). *Holy fools in Byzantium and beyond* (S. Franklin, Trans.). Oxford studies in Byzantium. Oxford: Oxford University Press.

Jaeger, W. (1943). *Paideia: The ideals of Greek culture* (G. Highet, Trans., Vol. II). New York: Oxford University Press.

Jaeger, W. (1973). *Paideia: The ideals of Greek culture* (G. Highet, Trans., Vol. I). New York: Oxford University Press.

Krell, D. F. (2016). *Ecstasy, catastrophe. Heidegger from being and time to the black notebooks*. New York: SUNY Press.

Krueger, D. (1996). *Symeon the holy fool: Leontius's life and the late antique city*. Berkeley, Los Angeles & London: University of California Press.

Lacan, J. (1993). *The seminar of Jacques Lacan. Book III 1955–1956* (J.-A. Miller, Ed.). London: Routledge.

Lacan, J. (2006). *Écrits. The first complete edition in English* (B. Fink, Trans.). New York & London: W. W. Norton & Company.

Lampe, G. W. H. (1961). *A patristic Greek lexicon*. Oxford: The Clarendon Press.

Lang, H. (1997). *Language and the unconscious. Lacan's hermeneutics of psychoanalysis* (T. Brockelman, Trans.). Atlantic Highlands, NJ: Humanities Press.

Laplanche, J. (1961). *Hölderlin et la question du père*. Paris: Presses Universitaires de France.

Lévy-Valensi, E. A. (1956). Vérité et langage du dialogue platonicien au dialogue psychoanalytique. *La Psychanalyse*, *1*, 257–274.

Lewy, H. (1929). *Sobria Ebrietas*. Untersuchungen zur Geschichte der antiken Mystik. Gliessen: Alfred Töplemann.

Linforth, M. (1946a). The corybantic rites in Plato. *University of California Publications in Classical Philology*, *XIII*(5), 121–162.

Linforth, M. (1946b). Telestic madness in Plato Phaedrus 244DE. *University of California Publications in Classical Philology*, *XIII*(6), 163–172.

Lossky, V. (1957). *The mystical theology of the Eastern church*. London: James Clarke and Co. Ltd.

Malherbe, A. J. (1970). Gentle as a nurse. The cynic background to I thess. ii. *Novum Testamentum*, *12*(2), 203–217.

Malingrey, A.-M. (1961). *"Philosophia". Étude d'un groupe de mots dans la literature grecque, des Présocratiques au ive siècle après J.-C.* Pars: Librairie C. Klincksieck.

Murray, G. (1912). *Four stages of Greek religion*. New York: Columbia University Press.

Nachmansohn, M. (1915). Freuds Libidotheorie verglichen mit Eroslehre Platos. *Internationale Zeitschrift für Ärzliche Psychoanalyse*, III Jahrgang, Heft 1, 65–83.

North, H. (2019). *Sophrosyne. Self-knowledge and Self-restraint in Greek literature*. St. Augustine, FL: Sophron Editor.

Oltramare, A. (1927). *Les origines de la diatribe romaine*. Lausanne: Payoll.

Patzer, A. (1987). *Der Historische Sokrates*. Darmstadt: Wissenschaftliche Buchgesellschaft.

Pfister, O. (1921). Plato als Vorlaufer der Psychoanalyse. *Internationale Zeitschrift für Psychoanalyse*, *VII*(3), 264–269.

Rottenberg, E. (2019). *For the love of psychoanalysis: The play of chance in Freud and Derrida*. Bronx: Fordham University Press.

Rydén, L. (Ed.). (1963). *Das Leben des heiligen Narren Symeon von Leontios von Neapolis*. Studia Graeca Upsaliensia (Vol. 4). Uppsala: University Library.

Santas, G. (1988). *Plato and Freud. Two theories of love*. Oxford: Basil Blackwell.

Schürmann, R. (2008). Heidegger's being and time. In S. Critchley, R. Schürmann, & S. Levine (Eds.), *On Heidegger's being and time* (pp. 56–131). London & New York: Routledge.

Sikes, E. E. (1931). *The Greek view of poetry*. London: Methuen and Co. Ltd.

Špidlík, T. (1963). Fous pour Christ. In *Dictionnaire de Spiritualité* (pp. XXXV–XXXVI, col. 752–761). Paris: Beauchesne.

Stok, F. (2007). Psychology. In C. W. Kallendorf (Ed.), *A companion to the classical tradition* (pp. 355–370). Oxford: Wiley-Blackwell.

Strunk, N. R. (n.d.). *Is the doctrine of the transcendentals viable today? Reflections on metaphysics and the doctrine of the transcendentals*. www.metaphysicalsociety.org/2011/Session%20VII.Strunk.pdf.

Tigerstedt, E. N. (1970). Furor poeticus: Poetic inspiration in Greek literature before Democritus and Plato. *Journal of the History of Ideas, 31*(2), 163–178.

Tsai, W.-D. (2018). On Heidegger's concept of poet. *Proceedings of the XXIII World Congress of Philosophy, 33*, 25–29.

Urbainczyk, T. (2002). *Theodoret of Cyrrhus*. The *bishop and the holy man*. Ann Arbor, MI: The University of Michigan Press.

Vanheule, S. (2017). Conceptualizing and treating psychosis: A Lacanian perspective: Conceptualizing and treating psychosis. *British Journal of Psychotherapy, 33*(3), 388–398.

Vicaire, P. (1963). Les Grecs et le mystère de l'inspiration poétique. *Bulletin de l'Association Guillaume Budé, 1*, 68–85.

Wasmuth, E. (2015). ὥσπερ οἱ κορυβαντιῶντες: The Corybantic Rites in Plato's dialogues. *The Classical Quarterly* (New Series) (65), 69–84.

Welborn, L. L. (2005). *Paul, the fool of Christ: A study of 1 Corinthians 1–4 in the comic-philosophical tradition*. London & New York: T and T Clark International.

Wensinck, A. J. (Trans.). (1923). *Mystic treatises by Isaac of Nineveh*. Amsterdam: Koninklijke Nederlandse Akademie van Wetenschappen.

Wickkister, B. L. (2008). *Asklepios, medicine, and the politics of healing in fifth-century Greece*. Baltimore: The John Hopkins University Press.

Chapter 6

Archetypal dimensions of expanded states

Tim Read

ABSTRACT: The traditional bio-psycho-social model of psyche is inadequate for our understanding of expanded states of consciousness such as reflected in psychedelic experiences and cases of spiritual emergency. I suggest that adding an archetypal perspective to produce a bio-psycho-socio-archetypal (BPSA) model gives us a more complete picture. I will begin with a description of a spiritual emergency before exploring the allegory of Plato's cave to offer an initial perspective of the territory that we may traverse in moving away from consensus reality. In this connection, I refer to the work of Stanislav Grof concerning the areas of psyche that become available to us in expanded states. I introduce the concept of archetypal penetrance and comment on the importance of attachment, early trauma, adverse life events and psychodynamic factors.

KEYWORDS: archetypal, Kundalini, perinatal, psychedelic, transpersonal

Christina felt like she had been hit by a miraculous but frightening force when she was giving birth to her first child as powerful and unfamiliar energies began to stream through her body. She shook uncontrollably, she felt electric tremors coursing through her, and she had visions of white light. The sensations settled quite quickly but recurred two years later when she was in labor with her second child. On this occasion, she was given a tranquilizing injection which confirmed her feeling that what had happened was a sign of illness and somehow shameful. The next such experience occurred a few years later, when she met a Hindu teacher who subsequently became her guru. She felt as though she had been "plugged into a high-voltage socket" (Grof C., 1990, p. 11), but this time it was accompanied by an intense and turbulent emotional release that challenged her worldview and her identity. Her crisis deepened after a car crash when she seemed to pass through an opaque curtain of death into a deep feeling of connection with everything in the universe. She thought she was going crazy and would be institutionalized.

In her search for healing, she met the man who was to become her husband, the psychiatrist Stanislav Grof. Her inner turmoil intensified but Grof recognized her symptoms as similar to those he had encountered in his therapeutic work with LSD. He reassured her that this was not irreversible psychosis but an important step in her psychospiritual journey – a spiritual emergency. Grof suggested that rather than resist the symptoms, she should allow herself to fully experience and move through them. This was an entirely new perspective for her, and she found that it was indeed a cleansing process and a crucial movement toward her healing and wholeness.

As Christina surrendered to her inner experience, she describes jolts of energy and a multitude of images such as monsters ripping her to shreds or disconnected probing eyes. She died many deaths, feeling that some were her own, and at other times assuming the role of historical figures who had died in difficult circumstances. At times, she would scream and roll on the floor with fear and pain – Grof supported her throughout. The worst of the crisis abated after five days, although she continued to experience emotional turbulence, visionary sequences, and strange energetic phenomena. She was left with a paradigm-changing realization:

> I was more than my physical body: I also had a vast spiritual self that had been there all the time waiting for me to discover it. Feeling that my potential was limitless, I recognised that my task in life was to clear away the personal restrictions that kept me from realising those possibilities.
>
> (Grof C., 1990, p. 16)

The Swiss psychiatrist C.G. Jung also experienced energetic phenomena and visions during his psychospiritual crisis triggered by his break with Sigmund Freud. Jung made a conscious decision to surrender to his unconscious processes in the service of enquiry, therapeutic endeavor, and personal growth. How could he help his patients if he did not explore the territory himself, he asked? Jung was convinced that Freud's theories, while valid, were only part of a bigger picture and that there was a deeper layer of psyche with a numinous tone and rich in symbolism that needed to be explored. But Jung was taken aback by the sheer difficulty of his task:

> I stood helpless before an alien world; everything in it seemed difficult and incomprehensible. I was living in a constant state of tension. . . . One thunderstorm followed another. My enduring these storms was a question of brute strength and from the beginning there was no doubt in my mind that I must find the meaning of what I was experiencing in these fantasies. When I endured these assaults from the unconscious I had the unswerving conviction that I was obeying a higher will and that feeling continued to uphold me until I had mastered the task.
>
> (Jung, 1963, p. 201)

The phenomenology of such psychospiritual crises cannot be understood with the prevailing psychiatric, psychological, or psychoanalytic models of mind.

We require additional maps while recognizing that multiple models and reference points are likely to be required for different people at different times in their journeys. There is a view that maps are misleading and that all that is required is support while nature takes its healing course. This may indeed be true while in the eye of the storm. But as the storm abates and the integrative process accelerates, it is helpful for journeyers and those who support them to have tools and guides to help them make sense of and integrate the fruits of their journey.

The model that I will outline can be termed bio-psycho-socio-archetypal (BPSA). While the bio-psycho-social model prevails in British psychiatry and will be familiar to many, I suggest the addition of an archetypal perspective with an emphasis on the primary colors of *meaning*, recognition of numinous states, and transpersonal experience. I use the term archetype here as a transpersonal construct that extends beyond the individual psyche and involves a deeper order linked by meaning. In this scheme of things, meaning could even be understood as a fifth dimension to add to our four-dimensional space-time construct. I will often use the term archetypal crisis instead of spiritual emergency, as it is not always clear to people undergoing such crises that there is a spiritual component. I will discuss the significance of the perinatal and transpersonal layers of psyche and how they relate to the experiences of Christina Grof, C.G. Jung, and others.

Models are simply models, and it requires skill and experience to use such tools to bring understanding to highly complex and multi-layered psychological states. Flexibility, humility, and compassion have to be in the forefront. An ideological preference for a particular model at the expense of a broader picture tends toward the reductionist, even fundamentalist, approaches that bedevil this field. Any discussion of spiritual emergency and an archetypal perspective in my view needs to be balanced by the recognition that for many people, a more medical model can also lead to emancipation from destabilizing symptoms. There are many for whom a diagnosis of, for example, bipolar disorder and the prescription of medication can be helpful. However, for people with the mindset of curiosity and the ability to tolerate some distress in the service of growth, the archetypal crisis/spiritual emergence model holds enormous potential for the healing of deep psychological wounds and for psychospiritual progress.

Plato's cave

Plato and his teacher Socrates are the founding fathers of our Western philosophical tradition. In his allegory of the cave (Figure 6.1), Plato gives us a coherent account of the mystical adventure, the hero's journey, the psychospiritual crisis (Waterfield, 1993). We can be sure that this was a story that had been honed by rigorous thought and Socratic dialogue, but it was also informed by deep experiential work. Many luminaries of the classical world, including Plato, attended

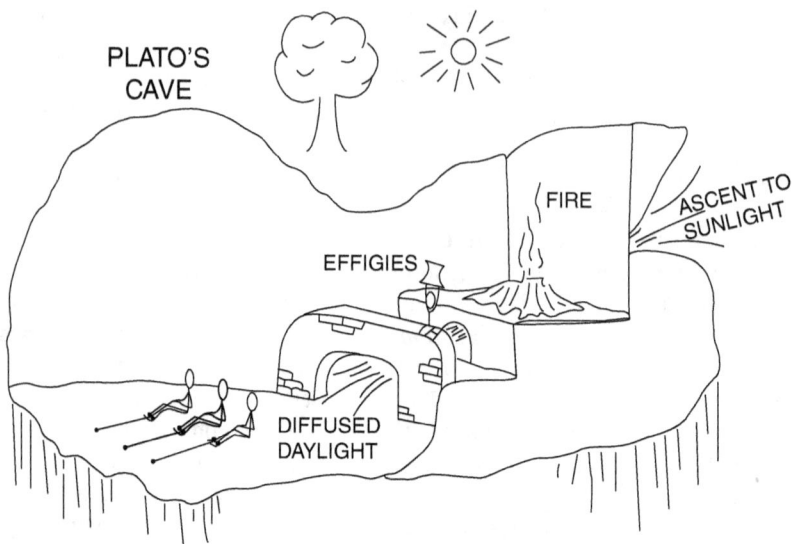

Figure 6.1 Plato's cave.

the Eleusinian mysteries where a psychedelic potion was taken in a ceremonial setting. Plutarch gives us a flavor of the rites of Eleusis as follows:

> Wandering astray in the beginning, tiresome wandering in circles, some frightening paths in darkness that lead nowhere. The before the end, all the terrible things – panic and shivering, sweat and amazement. And then some wonderful light comes to greet you, with sounds and dances, sacred words and holy views.
>
> (Burkert, 1983, p. 168)

Plato's allegory of the cave depicts humans who are chained in the depths of a cave so that they have no choice but to gaze at the projected images on the viewing screen represented by the back of the cave. This could be termed a state of *endarkenment*, where there is no sense of a greater scheme of things and the individual is completely invested in the world of illusion. There are two sources of light in the cave, the most obvious being the firelight that casts shadows of the effigies paraded before it to create flickering images. These images represent our consensus reality, which is an illusion created by the narratives forming our conditioning and molded by our cognitive structures. But there is also a trickle of light from the sun diffusing down the passageway to the world outside that represents a different form of consciousness entirely. Plato's sunlight could be compared to Huxley's Mind at Large:

> To make biological survival possible, Mind at Large has to be funneled through the reducing valve of the brain and nervous system. What comes out at the other end is a measly trickle of the kind of consciousness, which will help us to stay alive on the surface of this particular planet.
>
> (Huxley, 1954, pp. 12–13)

Plato describes the start of the emancipatory journey as our hero breaks free from the chains, turns toward the light and begins the ascent to the higher dimensional reality outside of the cave. He (for the Greek philosopher was inevitably male) has an encounter with the ego structures represented by the effigies, before emerging from the black and white environment of the cave to the indescribably richer and more colorful world outside. He may even enjoy a moment of cosmic union with the primary source represented by the sun. Then the enlightened being cautiously returns to the illusory world of the cave and uses his knowledge wisely for the benefit of the cave dwellers. In Plato's view, the numinous perspective gained by the journey was an essential tool for the task of the philosopher ruler.

Plato's allegory provides a possible model for thinking about the transformation of consciousness in expanded states and the way in which transpersonal elements of consciousness interact with our ego structures. I suggest that there are four distinct phases of this transformative journey: a three-phase ascent followed by the descent and return (Read, 2015, p. 106). A crisis may occur at each level of the journey, and in cases of spiritual emergency there may well be a crisis associated with each level simultaneously. The phases are as follows:

- Turning away from consensus reality
- Encounter with the personal unconscious
- Progression to archetypal and transpersonal elements
- Return

The ascent

The ascent has three phases: the turning away from consensus reality, the encounter with the unconscious, and the emergence of archetypal material. With an enquiring mindset and the right support system, the ascent may be undertaken intentionally; this reflecting a determination to lean into and learn from challenging experiences. There are a number of methods that can be adopted to pursue this goal, such as the ritual taking of a psychedelic substance, nondrug methods such as holotropic breathwork, meditation, or other forms of intense spiritual practice where the modern equivalent of the philosopher makes an intentional voyage into the deep psyche. Such a journey may suggest an intention to resolve trauma and heal psychological wounds, or there may be a more general purpose to open to the archetypal dimensions of the psyche, awaken to spirit, and return refreshed and renewed. It is above all an internal journey whereby stimuli from the outside world are heavily modified, often with blindfold and a music set. There is a high level of support from others and formal integration techniques after the return to everyday consciousness to make sure that the fruit of the journey is retained, rather than left to dissipate. The journeyer makes a full return to consensus reality and feels completely grounded by the time of return to the everyday world.

In archetypal crisis, the process is triggered involuntarily in an individual who is typically totally unprepared and ill equipped for the challenge. The onset of the psychological turbulence is perceived as disturbing and dangerous. The instinct of the person and their support systems aims at symptom suppression, and it is unusual for there to be any concept that symptoms may suggest the beginning of a healing journey. The turning away from consensus reality usually (but not always) has an environmental trigger. The trigger may be an obvious life event that will typically have a powerful resonance with a previous unresolved trauma. Sometimes the trigger will resonate with something that lies so deep in the unconscious that although it may have a profound effect, the nature of the wound underlying this may remain hidden from our conscious understanding.

Returning to Plato's allegory, in archetypal crises, there are often difficulties at multiple levels of the cave combined with a failure of the return journey. As the ego defenses represented by the metaphorical chains fall away, he is increasingly exposed to his psychological wounds; some of the traumas causing these wounds may be obvious and accessible to memory, while other traumas will have their origin in preverbal development and will remain mysterious. I use the term trauma broadly; the traumas will range from normal developmental wounds that have not been fully processed to more obvious emotional and perhaps physical traumas. This uncovering may open up the landscape of depression, devastation, and hope-lessness – the dark night of the soul. The biographical material that starts coming to the surface becomes suffused with archetypal intensity – and this sometimes carries significant risk.

As the process develops, it is as though the journeyer is lost in transit in Plato's cave system, in emotional contact with a multitude of psychological wounds that are at the same time undergoing archetypal intensification – this being symbolized by the increased light from fire and sun. In elevated mood states, the level of trauma and conditioning may be bypassed altogether with a leap into the archetypal territory outside the cave. This experience can be intoxicating in its richness and color, and feel pregnant with promise. Everything is connected; there are synchronicities, energetic downloads, psychic experiences, and spiritual awakening. There may even be the loss of ego boundaries with dissolution into the universal consciousness.

In archetypal crisis, the trajectory of ascent and return tends to be lost and the journeyer cannot easily return to consensus reality. So a situation develops where a person experiences a highly problematic encounter with unconscious process that is undergoing archetypal amplification, resulting in increased intensity of meaning. There may be the added complexity of transpersonal experience, which is represented in Plato's allegory by the extra-dimensional territory of the world outside the cave. This is complicated further by the consequences of failure in the return, with the person being unable to function adequately in everyday life. The longer a person stays in such territory, the more likely it is that support systems and behavior become disorganized. Such secondary psychosocial complications perpetuate the crisis and the experience may be interpreted as illness. Encounters with mental health services are often seen as unhelpful and can be deeply traumatizing, especially if coercion is employed. Rather than being given a message of hope and healing, the person is likely to feel shamed and stigmatized. In such circumstances, the possibility of emergence and psychospiritual growth becomes limited; indeed, there is a significant risk of personality, behavior, and social function becoming lastingly organized around this dysfunctional position.

Archetypal penetrance

Archetypes flow through us; they are expressed through the hardware that is our body, our nervous system, and our sense organs. If we are indeed influenced by an archetypal ocean with tides, currents, waves, and undertows, then this may be more active – or *penetrant* – in some people than others and we may be more receptive to different archetypal flavors at different times of life. It is often observed that mysticism and madness have a common origin, and I suggest that this is due to a shared genetic predisposition to *high archetypal penetrance* (HAP) states (Read, 2019). This may result in an archetypal crisis, or it may predispose us to a more creative or spiritual state.

The advantages conferred by functional HAP states in society would explain the persistence in the population of dysfunctional HAP states that have become defined as mental illness. This constitutional predisposition to a broader range of conscious experience is enhanced by multiple risk factors that raise vulnerability to archetypal crisis. Some of these factors will also predispose to poor outcome. Such risk factors include problematic attachment patterns, adverse childhood experience, a family history of psychosis, social instability, personality disorder, and substance use. The point that I want to emphasize here is that a vicious circle can easily arise between constitutional vulnerability and environmental challenges, between nature and lack of nurture.

The nature of the archetype is inherently difficult to define. Archetypes are the great flavors of meaning; we used to call them the many names of the gods. Usually, the range of meaning that we experience is held within certain limits by our cognitive structures so that we can fulfill our daily tasks. In the same way that our ears and eyes only interpret a small range of available frequencies and wavelengths, our brain regulates the degree of meaning available to us. But in expanded states, our perception and range of meaning is enhanced and we move further into the numinous spectrum. The biological mechanism whereby this occurs has yet to be clarified, but recent research into the mode of action of psychedelic substances suggests that the default mode network in the brain may be involved in this process (Carhart-Harris et al., 2016).

Sometimes, the degree of archetypal penetrance is overwhelming and the amplification of meaning may cause a crisis as hitherto repressed psychological material floods the psyche. As Marie Louise Von Franz (1975) states: "when shadow projections arise from the archetypal psyche, insights come with almost insuperable difficulties" (p. 247). From this perspective, acute psychiatric disorders occur when there is a failure of the homeostatic mechanisms that normally maintain archetypal penetrance within a comfortable range. The morbid fear associated with paranoid states, the excitement and amplification of manic states, the loathing and constriction of severe depression, and the imminence of catastrophe found in post-traumatic stress disorder, all have an awe-filled quality that could be called numinous. This numinous quality is the fundamental characteristic of archetypal experience and imbues the crisis with overwhelming power. The term *numinous* is derived from the Latin word *numen*, which is usually translated as "divine presence" and implies a strong religious or spiritual quality. By definition, a numinous experience always involves a sense of the sacred. The German theologian Rudolf Otto (1923) described the numinous as the principle that underlies all religion, a mystery that both terrified and fascinated at the same time.

Otto defines the term sacred or holy as an *overplus* of meaning. In a numinous state, meaning is amplified so that the tone and resonance of meaning becomes overwhelming and magnetic. The crucial point about the idea of the numinous is its bivalence having both dark and light manifestations. It can be beautiful or dreadful, and the literature of religious experience abounds in references to the pains and terrors overwhelming those who have come, too suddenly, face to face with some manifestation of the numinous. Crucially, Otto describes how incomplete or partial forms of numinous experience can have a nightmarish primitive quality with an abrupt and capricious character, but this crude stage with its ominous tone has the potential to be transcended as the numen reveals itself and the process unfolds, eventually becoming integrated by the more rational elements of consciousness.

In archetypal crisis or high archetypal penetrance states, it is an article of faith that ominous mood states will eventually recede, that there is a teleological pull toward the resolution of psychological trauma. This has been likened to the tendency of physical wounds to heal, although of course this depends on the severity of the wound. For emotional wounds such as bereavement, the passage of time may be sufficient, but for deeper, more complex wounds, it may be that a crucial ingredient for resolution is to not only be open to psychological experience but to actively intensify, explore and work with it – a proactive and supported process of engagement with deep psyche. To do this, a positive mindset is required, but even with such an outlook this is a daunting process. Christina Grof and C.G. Jung both surrendered to their inner processes, were well supported and worked hard on the integration, but it took years for their symptoms to resolve.

The intentional intensification of symptoms would be a radical change for psychiatry where usual practice is to suppress them as meaningless epiphenomena of mental illness. We have very little research evidence as to what may be the outcome of intensification practice. Stanislav Grof (1975) used LSD psychotherapy in a specialized unit for psychiatric inpatients suffering from chronic and severe neurotic conditions in the 1950s and 1960s when LSD assisted treatment seemed to be the cutting edge of modern psychiatric practice. The LSD treatment allowed for intensification of symptoms and was supported throughout by integrative psychotherapy. I am not suggesting that people in archetypal crisis should be treated with psychedelics, but that the course of LSD psychotherapy and the way in which it is supported may provide a useful model to inform work with people in naturally occurring archetypal crisis.

In Grof's LSD psychotherapy unit, the treatment program typically lasted one year. The general trajectory of the clinical course of these patients supported Otto's prediction that the ominous tone resolves with repeated exposure and the numen does indeed reveal itself. In the course of LSD treatment, the patients typically spent the early sessions revisiting and processing events that had occurred in their lives and that still held a strong emotional charge. This was followed by a complex stage that seemed to transcend their biographical memories with themes of psychospiritual death and rebirth. Sometime this was followed by sessions with more transpersonal content, even experiences of cosmic unity (Plato's sun). The process was accompanied by clinical improvement, an increased sense of well-being, and changed attitudes toward death. It became clear to the researchers that the process paralleled historical descriptions of spiritual initiations in various cultures (Grof, 1975, p. 204).

The complex and the COEX

One of the features of an archetypal crisis is the conflation of biographical trauma with transpersonal material and the manner in which this is intensified by archetypal amplification. Some of the biographical material may be obvious and relate to trauma that is accessible to conscious memory. But what makes the process so confusing and difficult to navigate is that often the emerging material does not map onto conscious experience. The Jungian concept of the complex offers a structure of the psyche that gathers together similar feeling-toned elements. The richness and variety of complexes are major determinants of personality and unresolved complexes may exert unconscious, maladaptive influence on our thoughts, feelings, and behavior. We may feel familiar with the superficial layers of complex emotional states that resonate with abandonment, loss, envy, desire, anxiety, hope, or despair, to name a few. But the roots of our complexes are organized by early experiences that lie outside conscious memory. It is this primitive, germinative layer of our psyche with a powerful theme of annihilatory anxiety – death and rebirth – that forms the nucleus of our key complexes.

In his work with expanded states of consciousness, Grof (1975) found that people in these states tend to move readily between different octaves of meaning. Such expanded states facilitate the navigation of complexes. Grof made an important observation that an emotional state that seems primarily related to a childhood experience may, in an LSD session or spontaneous spiritual emergency, change to become an experience that has a very different quality – this being characterized by themes of life and death that do not relate to anything they can remember having happened to them. This may in turn progress to an archetypal experience with a mythic or dreamlike quality. Grof considered that the deepest layer of emotional experience, the very core of the complex, lay in perinatal experience – the trauma of our birth. He coined the term "system of condensed experience," or COEX system to incorporate this defining perinatal trauma.

I think that one of the fundamental characteristics of archetypal crisis is that our various traumas and historic unresolved issues constellate together according to the meaning tone of that trauma. Meaning is primary – so in order to make sense of the experience and integrate it, the attention to meaning has to be paramount. What gives the COEX its often terrifying or confusing quality is the progression from biographical material that we can easily remember to those preverbal formative experiences of birth and infancy. These early experiences – and especially the perinatal trauma, with its resonance with life and death – may act as a portal to transpersonal experiences, which often add more fuel to the crisis.

Different people will have a different number and flavor of COEX systems and each COEX system will have a characteristic relationship to psychological defenses. In his work with psychiatric inpatients using LSD, Grof (1975) found that a COEX system would often be revisited in successive sessions until it had been resolved and the patient would access new material with different emotions and meaning in the next series of sessions. Usually, experiences from later in life lie in the more accessible superficial layers of the COEX systems, but the core of the COEX derives from earliest experience.

The concept of the COEX helps us to understand the relationship between the different layers of psyche. Intense mental states cannot be understood according to just one level or model of psyche; rather, there is a sliding scale between the different levels exhibiting the same meaning tone. Thus, people with a psychodynamic structure predisposing to certain feeling states will be more likely to experience those feeling states with numinous intensity in high penetrance archetypal states. Turning this around, it seems likely that high archetypal penetrance states may offer an opportunity to access and resolve some of the unrecognized psychodynamics that may be problematic for us.

Preverbal trauma in the postnatal period

I consider it likely that archetypal crisis inevitably brings us into contact with preverbal trauma. This raises very challenging and powerful feelings that lie beyond memory and which are difficult to think about and articulate. Infantile events such as early disruption to feeding and attachment patterns leave powerful undertows that can play out in a variety of ways. Such early trauma increases vulnerability but probably also enhances capacity for resilience in those who are able to flourish.

There are some early traumas that are probably common to all of us, such as the experience of hunger with accompanying feelings of dis-ease, needs not being met, abandonment, rejection and ultimately a profound anxiety about survival. The raw and overwhelming feelings of hunger in the early postnatal state would be experienced as an assault by an external force, and these unbearable feelings are disowned and projected onto an external object (usually the mother) which then becomes identified with that feeling. The Kleinian school of psychoanalysis has labeled this the paranoid-schizoid position, and the baby's defense is one of projective identification (Klein, 1959).

The other side of this dynamic is the love that is projected on to the mother as a good object when the baby feels well fed and happy. Thus, our earliest way of understanding the world expresses a profound split between the all-good object and the all-bad object. The way in which this common experience is metabolized and becomes a template for future experiences of adversity varies enormously. For most of us, the containing aspects of maternal function bring us to a position where we can accommodate both good and bad versions of the same person – Klein terms this the depressive position. But if we are stressed or anxious, any of us may collapse into the default position of the paranoid-schizoid.

The psychiatrist Rob Charles gives a personal account of the onset of paranoid ideation and auditory hallucinations around puberty that seemed, with the benefit of hindsight, to have roots in prolonged starvation in infancy due to his mother's illness. He was the boy who was marked out by being different, the boy who emitted a rank odor. He was beginning to think that his mother may be doing something malign to him, perhaps putting something on his clothes. But the realization that this could not be possible marked the beginning of recovery:

> This was the turning point – my mother did love me, there could be no doubt of that. So I start to turn over in my mind the tantalising possibility that there was something the matter with my mind rather than my body. There are a number of bifurcation points in my story where I think matters could have got much worse. If I had not felt secure in my mother's love, if my home situation had been less secure, I suspect my thinking would have become more paranoid, my behaviour more bizarre and I would probably have become a psychiatric patient with everything that flows from that.
>
> (Evans & Read, 2020, p. 196)

Some people have the paranoid position as a dominant structure in their psyche. This state of mind has also been termed the fundamentalist position (Stokoe, 2019), and it is particularly obvious in extreme political groups where the political struggle is seen as a battle between light and dark, there is an assault by malign forces who conspire against you, and there is an idyll, a Golden Age which is being denied. In the spiritual emergency field, similar dynamics can sometimes be observed with the conviction that all psychiatry is bad, that the medical hierarchy and big pharma conspire against people with spiritual awakenings who are being denied enlightenment and maintained in a stupefied state by inappropriate medication and neglect.

In individuals, the significance of the paranoid position is multifold. It is a common bedrock of experience that we are likely to access in intense mental states. Usually it is transient and will respond to supportive measures. But some people will have difficulty withdrawing their projections from the external world. In such cases, they will struggle to understand their experience as an inner one. Their symptoms may become chronic and impermeable.

Death, rebirth, and the perinatal psyche

Stanislav Grof has delineated the importance of the perinatal process in the developing psyche. A full description of this work lies beyond the scope of this chapter, but interested readers will find rich food for thought in Grof's seminal book *Realms of the Human Unconscious* (1975). Grof introduces the perinatal layer as follows:

> The basic characteristics of perinatal experience and their central focus are the problems of biological birth, physical pain and agony, aging, disease and decrepitude, dying and death. Inevitably the shattering encounter with these critical aspects of human existence and the deep realisation of the frailty and impermanence of man as a biological creature is accompanied by an agonising existential crisis.
>
> (Grof, 1975, p. 95)

Grof's fundamental insight concerning the perinatal layer of psyche is that it is so rich, so complex, and so viscerally powerful that it acts as a template for much of our subsequent psychological development and is a fertile ground for psychopathology. Grof found that at its deepest level, all COEX systems have a perinatal component which needs to be accessed and allowed to flow into some form of resolution. The perinatal material is experienced in an archetypal manner as it occurred before the formation of ego structures or defenses. This archetypal quality with its intense and transgressive nature explains why this layer of psyche so often acts as a portal to transpersonal experience.

Grof reports that in expanded states of consciousness, people often experience moving beyond the level of memories from childhood and infancy, and encountering emotions and physical sensations of extreme intensity that hold a strange mixture of themes of birth and death. These included images, emotions and physical experiences that seem related to the birth process itself.

Looking at the birth process from the perspective of the baby, things start in the serenity of the womb, but the earthquake of the onset of labor disrupts this unitive state and paradise is decisively lost. There follows the life-or-death struggle through the birth canal and the exhausted deliverance into an alien world with all its sound, fury, and separation. These four very distinct meaning states comprise Grof's basic perinatal matrices (BPM).

- The first perinatal matrix (BPM 1) is the resting state that lasts until the onset of the contractions of labor. The baby develops peacefully in the amniotic sac with her entire needs being met by the encompassing and nourishing mother. Occasionally this resting state becomes poisonous, perhaps due to medication, toxins, or lack of oxygen.
- The second perinatal matrix (BPM 2) is the physical onset of labor where the uterus contracts against a closed cervix. There is no available exit, so this state involves an experience of constriction, entrapment, and fear; the baby faces death.
- The third perinatal matrix (BPM 3) represents the physical process of movement out of the constricted uterus through the opening cervix followed by the "life-or-death struggle" through the birth canal. The infant's body is subject to great forces of a constricting, twisting, pulsing nature. But there is movement and the possibility of salvation.
- The fourth perinatal matrix (BPM 4) is the birth, the emergence into the light, the first intake of breath and the recovery phase for mother and baby. The ordeal is over, and they can meet each other for the first time in the outside world. But this can seem a hostile and irrevocably changed environment. The primal unity with mother is lost forever. It can feel more like a death than a birth.

The significance of the perinatal layer of psyche lies is its extraordinary duration and level of violence, both on an emotional and a physical level. It is not surprising that it is so often experienced as a tortured death. Very few people will have experienced anything approaching this level of physical violence and annihilatory anxiety in the remainder of their lives.

One possible explanation for the dramatic symptoms reported by Christina Grof with the multiple death sequences is that it contains a re-enactment of the birth process. In Christina's case, it may be that her initial crisis was triggered by her going into labor with her first baby and this had a resonance with her own unresolved perinatal trauma. It may also be that her archetypal penetrance was raised by her years of yoga practice, which made her more vulnerable to archetypal crisis.

In the archetypal states that correspond to the perinatal journey, the first perinatal matrix involving good-womb experiences would equate to oceanic feelings of bliss and cosmic unity. If a toxic womb state develops before birth, this may equate to feeling poisoned or paranoid. The second perinatal matrix typically involves feelings of profound hopelessness, existential despair, insuperable forces ranged against one, and the inevitability of death. This is the territory of the "bad trip" after the paradise of the first matrix is lost. The third perinatal matrix is the archetypal hero's journey, the call to arms, the tumultuous and perilous struggle. The fourth perinatal matrix holds themes of triumph, fortuitous escape from danger, revolution, decompression and expansion of space, radiant light, and color.

In expanded states and especially in archetypal crisis, the mental experiences do not follow the sequence of the birth process. Instead, the most emotionally charged fragments of experience are brought to conscious awareness and content may incorporate aspects of any basic perinatal matrix. An archetypal crisis, as opposed to a psychedelic journey, allows a prolonged exposure to highly challenging mental experiences. As Deborah Martin puts it:

> The difference between a bad trip and the start of a spiritual emergency is that one is a dark alley, the other a labyrinth. One a snarling dog, the other a wild predator. One a fall down a well, the other a tumble into a black hole.
>
> (Evans & Read, 2020, p. 3)

Stephen Fitzpatrick describes a crisis developing after intense spiritual practice that I suggest has resonance with the dislocation of the fourth perinatal matrix when there is death to a familiar way of being:

> Something was wrong, really, deeply wrong. It wasn't a familiar kind of wrong. . . . Then came the initial realisation. The wrongness isn't in the details, it's in everything because I am dead, I have died. . . . I had been alive and now I am dead. This wasn't a thought. There was nothing speculative about it. It was a direct perception.
>
> (Evans & Read, 2020, p. 76)

Fitzpatrick made a recovery from his crisis with the assistance of psychotherapy and Qi Gong, but a year afterwards during a first trip to Morocco he had a recurrence, the description of which exhibits a resonance with the second perinatal matrix:

> someone or something is releasing sharks into me . . . waves of shattering, tearing rending from head to toe tear me apart . . . an unstoppable school of night sea monsters heading for my torso, my head. . . . I am going to die. . . . I sense the background presence of two figures, mantis-like shadow puppets picking at each others' eyes, screaming and shouting. They are the orchestraters. This is their chamber of horrors . . . the bloody chamber.
>
> (Evans & Read, 2020, p. 82)

The archetypal crisis may be triggered by psychedelic drugs, especially if taken in unsupportive settings or with inadequate integration. The philosopher Jules Evans describes the aftermath of an ayahuasca retreat in Peru and the shock of leaving the safety of the temple and the abrupt return to "the dirty, smelly, noisy town of Iquitos":

> Time stretched nauseatingly. Why weren't the people around me questioning this endless wait? Because they weren't real. I felt like I was in a computer game, and the next level was failing to load. The other people didn't react or notice this glitch, because they were dumb non-playable characters in a computer game. I thought, I'm going to be stuck here forever, stuck between levels.
>
> No, I was dead, and in some ghastly afterlife. These ghoulish ferry-men were Charon and his crew, taking us across the Styx. I stared at the water bleakly. This is not how I imagined the afterlife.
>
> (Evans & Read, 2020, p. 50)

Resolution involves catharsis, identified by Josef Breuer (Breuer, 1974) as fundamental to the talking cure. Breuer's key insight was that traumatic experiences can be repressed and continue to reside in the unconscious, motivating behavior and re-emerge as symptoms unless they can be remembered and spoken about. But in expanded states, the process of catharsis may be more complex and mysterious than simply talking. Catharsis may occur on an emotional level or a physical level; it may be ineffable and integrative methods other than words may need to be deployed. Both Jung and the Grofs found that more artistic methods of expression were invaluable.

Transpersonal experience

Many people report anomalous experiences during spiritual emergencies that cannot be accounted for by the prevailing models of mind favored by the medical and scientific establishment. On the other side of the argument, there is evidence supporting the existence of a transmissive aspect of mind – that mental life has a field effect. Psi, a term used in parapsychology research, denotes anomalous processes of information or energy transfer; an interaction between consciousness and the physical world. Psi includes processes such as telepathy, precognition, psychokinesis, and other forms of extrasensory perception that are currently unexplained in terms of known physical or biological mechanisms. The term psi is purely descriptive; it does not imply that such phenomena are paranormal and it does not make conclusions about their underlying mechanisms (Bem & Honorton, 1994). Rupert Sheldrake (2012, p. 239) suggests that psi should be considered a perfectly natural phenomenon that academic science has not yet accepted or incorporated into mainstream thinking.

Christina Grof had a number of synchronicities, while Jung reported precognitive dreams and communications with spirits. Jules Evans found that immediately after his ayahuasca retreat he had a strong sense of connection to the other people at the temple and "felt quite psychic, as if I could tell what people were going to say milliseconds before they said it" (Evans & Read, 2020, p. 77). This heightened degree of connectivity is characteristic of the archetypal territory outside of Plato's cave, and will be familiar to people who have been on retreats or similar where a group of people spend some time together in expanded states of consciousness.

Of course, opinion is deeply divided between those who consider that there are elements of consciousness that are independent of brain and synapse and those who hold that consciousness can only exist as a result of brain activity. I suggest that even if one accepts that genuine transpersonal experiences occur (such as synchronicity), there may be alterations in brain function that not only increase the likelihood of such experiences but also may make it more difficult for such experiences to be integrated. In an agitated and distressed state, any transpersonal phenomena may add to the confusion and fuel the crisis.

When people have emerged from their crisis, they may be able to communicate such experiences in a lucid and thoughtful manner. But often, people in crisis may lack coherence in their communication and transpersonal experience may be conflated with traumatic material relating to ego structures, which compounds the difficulty in making sense of it. Indeed, Plato described the difficulties of the return in that the person returning from beyond the cave would be dazzled by the sunlight, would struggle to readjust to the gloom of the cave, and would be slow and backward at recognizing the shadows. Plato suggests that his comrades would not only scorn him for his impairment of function but would also be deeply unimpressed by anything that he had to tell them about where he had been and what he had discovered.

If the reality of synchronicities is accepted, rather than dismissed as ideas of reference, it implies that meaning has united an internal experience and an external event. Such realizations do not support the notion of consciousness as entirely limited to the bony confines of the skull and tend to be paradigm changing. Indeed, a major synchronicity is a numinous event that has changed the worldview of people such as Augustine, Jung, Koestler, and Joseph Campbell (Read, 2019, pp. 66–67).

As Von Franz puts it: "the most impressive thing about synchronistic occurrences, the thing that really constitutes their numinosity, is that in them the duality of soul and matter seems to be eliminated" (Von Franz, 1975, p. 247). They are therefore an empirical indication of the ultimate unity of all existence. For Tarnas (2006), a "synchronicity serves a definite purpose, impelling the psyche toward a more complete psychological and spiritual realization of the individual personality" (p. 53). This is a crucial distinction; a synchronicity is growth oriented, although to achieve this growth requires care, thought, and integration.

In psychiatric practice, it is not uncommon for people in excited states to over-attribute meaning to unconnected events. It may seem to them as though there are synchronicities everywhere. This may amount to *delusions of reference*, a pathological state where, for example, a person may feel that every passing car registration number is imbued with a personal meaning. Clearly, such states are dysfunctional and do not have integrative or growth potential, at least in the short term – but psychiatrists do need to be able to distinguish between genuine syn-chronicities and psychosis, and avoid treating all unusual phenomena as mental illness.

I do not suggest that all anomalous experience is the result of transpersonal factors rather than abnormal brain function, merely that this is a legitimate area for further discussion. The key to managing archetypal crisis is that the unusual experiences have meaning and growth potential, and are not simply pathological symptoms that should be dismissed as meaningless.

Conclusion

What are we to make of the intense and unfamiliar energies, the electric tremors described by Christina Grof? These phenomena are mysterious and can feel totally overwhelming for those who experience them. Indeed, Christina Grof found it so difficult to tolerate these energies that she describes the development of an alcohol problem as a result (Grof, 1990, p. 100). Ram Dass (1989) likened the inrush of energy to an overdose of electricity: "If you were a toaster, it would be like stick-ing your plug into 220 volts rather than 110 volts" (p. 180).

Such energetic phenomena are described in spiritual awakenings, archetypal crises, and psychedelic states. The impact of these experiences is heavily influ-enced by set and setting. In highly supportive settings such as holotropic breath-work retreats, these states are usually experienced as helpful. On the other hand, patients in the emergency room who had arrived in stressful circumstances would frequently describe to me somatic sensations of heat, flutterings, or pressure that were deeply disturbing and frightening for them.

A number of explanatory models for such symptoms have been advanced, including abnormal brain function, an energetic experience from an external transpersonal source, or an energetic experience from an inner source. Such an inner source may be a somatic release relating to early physical trauma such as the birth process. There may be elements of each of these, but I suggest that the Kun-dalini model described in what follows is particularly useful, as it has resonance with the cleansing process that people often feel they are undergoing when they experience such phenomena in a supported setting.

In Hindu culture, Kundalini awakening develops slowly in the context of spir-itual practice, allowing a gradual adjustment to the lowering of ego defenses and opening to the deeper layers of mind. Traditionally, the full process of Kundalini awakening takes at least three years for advanced practitioners. Experiences with similar characteristics in the West can be much shorter, but more problematic. The American psychiatrist and ophthalmologist Lee Sannella (1989) distinguishes a *physio-kundalini syndrome*, which has the characteristics and sensations of the archetypal inrush without the complete integrated process of a full Kundalini awakening. Sannella found that such people did not have the first-rank symptoms that psychiatrists are taught to recognize as characteristic of schizophrenia and that physical sensations such as heat, electrical sensations, fluttering, vibrations, or spontaneous movements are common.

Sannella describes the kundalini process in metaphorical terms:

> Just as an intense flow of water through a thick rubber pipe will cause the hose to whip around violently, while the same flow through a fire hose would hardly be noticed, so also does the flow of Kundalini through obstructed "channels" within the body or mind cause motions of those areas until the obstructions have been washed out and the channels "widened." The terms channel, widen, blocks, must be taken metaphorically. They may not refer to actual structures, dimensions and processes, but be only useful analogies for understanding this model of Kundalini. The actual process is undoubtedly much more subtle and complex.
>
> (Sannella, 1989, p. 104)

Such somatic sensations are an important hallmark of archetypal crisis and strongly indicate the need of an approach of supporting this natural process toward resolution. Providing that risk can be safely managed, medication is contraindicated as it runs the danger of blocking a healing process, thus preventing the discharge and working through of important psychological material. Indeed, this would be an ideal opportunity to deploy the best model of set, setting, and integration to harness a powerful opportunity for healing and growth. The strategy would be to encourage a mindset of curiosity and inquiry, to tolerate distress in the service of growth while providing a safe, gentle, and compassionate environment and appropriate psychotherapy to deepen understanding and manage a fruitful return. In order to fulfill this task, the therapist needs to have thorough knowledge of the psychological landscape and, like Plato's philosopher, to have benefited from his or her own adventure in consciousness.

The approach I have described is contrary to the usual psychiatric method of symptom suppression, whereby unusual experiences are considered pathological and meaningless. People working in mental health services usually have a strong sense of vocation but are not trained to tolerate and work with their clients' psychological distress with the aim of finding meaning in symptoms to promote healing, growth, and health. It is difficult to see this changing unless radical action is taken, such as legislation to allow for medication-free treatment models.

References

Bem, D. J., & Honorton, C. (1994). Does psi exist? Replicable evidence for an anomalous process of information transfer. *Psychological Bulletin, 115,* 4–18.

Breuer, J. (1974). *Studies on hysteria.* Harmondsworth: Penguin Books.

Burkert, W. (1983). *The anthropology of ancient Greece.* Berkeley, CA.

Carhart-Harris, R., Muthukumaraswamy, S., Roseman, L., Kaelen, M., et al. (2016). *Neural correlates of the LSD experience revealed by multimodal neuroimaging.* https://doi.org/10.1073/pnas.1518377113.

Charles, R. (2020). The boy who stank to high heaven. In J. Evans & T. Read (Eds.), *Breaking open: Finding a way through spiritual emergency.* London: Aeon Books.

Dass, R. (1989). Promises and pitfalls of the spiritual path. In S. Grof & C. Grof (Eds.), *Spiritual emergency: When personal transformation becomes a crisis.* New York: Penguin Putnam.

Evans, J. (2020). The in-between place. In J. Evans & T. Read (Eds.), *Breaking open: Finding a way through spiritual emergency.* London: Aeon Books.

Evans, J., & Read, T. (2020). *Breaking open: Finding a way through spiritual emergency.* London: Aeon Books.

Grof, S. (1975). *Realms of the human unconscious.* New York: Viking.

Grof, C. (1990). *The stormy search for the self.* New York: Penguin Putnam.

Grof, S., & Grof, C. (Eds.). (1989). *Spiritual emergency: When personal transformation becomes a crisis.* New York: Penguin Putnam.

Huxley, A. (1954). *Doors of perception.* London: Flamingo.

Jung, C.G. (1963). *Memories, dreams, reflections.* London: Routledge & Kegan Paul.

Klein, M. (1959). Our adult world and its roots in infancy. *Human Relations,* 12.

Otto, R. (1923). *The idea of the holy.* Oxford: Oxford University Press.

Read, T. (2015). Archaidelics. In R. Dickens & T. Read (Eds.), *Out of the shadows: A cornucopia from the psychedelic press.* London: Muswell Hill Press.

Read, T. (2019). *Walking shadows: Archetype and psyche in crisis and growth.* London: Aeon Books.

Sannella, L. (1989). Kundalini: Classical and clinical. In S. Grof & C. Grof (Eds.), *Spiritual emergency: When personal transformation becomes a crisis.* New York: Penguin Putnam.

Sheldrake, R. (2012). *The science delusion.* London: Coronet.

Stokoe, P. (2019). Where have all the adults gone? In D. Morgan (Ed.), *The unconscious in social and political life* (pp. 1–25). London: Phoenix.

Tarnas, R. (2006). *Cosmos and psyche: Intimations of a new world view.* New York: Viking.

Von Franz, M-L. (1975) *C.G. Jung: His myth in our time.* Toronto, ON: Inner City Books.

Waterfield, R. (1993). *Plato: The republic.* Oxford: Oxford University Press.

Chapter 7

Reconceptualizing John Nash's psychosis

A Lacanian perspective

Derek Hook

ABSTRACT: This chapter offers a Lacanian perspective on the psychosis of John Nash Jr., the Nobel Prize-winning mathematician whose life was recounted in Sylvia Nasar's celebrated biography *A Beautiful Mind* (1998), which was the basis of Ron Howard's Oscar-winning film (2001) of the same name. I begin by offering a critical engagement with an existing psychoanalytic account of Nash's life, namely that advanced in several papers by Donald Capps, who alleges, among other things, that Nash was a highly narcissistic personality. I take Capps's work to be indicative of a series of questionable assumptions that an overly stylized – if not derivative – form of psychoanalytic explanation routinely engenders in its descriptions of psychosis. Conceptualizations of this sort invariably approach psychosis in ways which are, if not explicitly, then implicitly devaluing of psychotic subjects. Such accounts are, as a general rule, strongly focused on the cognitive and psychological deficits of people with psychosis. They are, in addition, powerfully juvenilizing inasmuch as they tirelessly reiterate notions of regression, fixation and primal defenses. The result of this conceptualization, I argue, is that psychotic subjects are demoted to what is effectively a second-class order of subjectivity. Both by critiquing the explanations mobilized by Capps and by advancing a Lacanian conceptualization of certain of Nash's psychotic features, I hope to show both that a Lacanian orientation is not grounded in such a devaluing framework of ideas and that it opens up a series of enabling – indeed, emancipatory – perspectives on psychotic suffering.

KEYWORDS: delusions, narcissism, Name-of-the-Father, psychotic structure, the symbolic order.

Introduction

This chapter offers a Lacanian perspective on the psychosis of John Nash Jr., the Nobel Prize-winning mathematician whose life was recounted in Sylvia Nasar's celebrated biography *A Beautiful Mind* (1998), which was the basis of Ron Howard's Oscar-winning film (2001) of the same name. I begin by offering a critical engagement with an existing psychoanalytic account of Nash's life, namely that advanced in several papers by Donald Capps (2003, 2004a, 2004b, 2005), who alleges, among other things, that "Nash was a highly narcissistic personality" (2004b, p. 289). I take Capps's work to be indicative of a series of questionable assumptions that an overly stylized – if not derivative – form of psychoanalytic explanation routinely engenders in its descriptions of psychosis. Conceptualizations of this sort invariably approach psychosis in ways which are, if not explicitly, then implicitly devaluing of psychotic subjects. Such accounts are, as a general rule, strongly focused on the cognitive and psychological deficits of psychotic persons. They are, in addition, powerfully juvenilizing inasmuch as they tirelessly reiterate notions of regression, fixation and primal defenses (Sass, 2017). The result of this conceptualization, I argue, is that psychotic subjects are demoted to what is effectively a second-class order of subjectivity. Both by critiquing the explanations mobilized by Capps and by advancing a Lacanian conceptualization of certain of Nash's psychotic features, I hope to show both that a Lacanian orientation is not grounded in such a devaluing framework of ideas and that it opens up a series of enabling – indeed, emancipatory – perspectives on psychotic suffering.

Psychoanalytic devaluations: a critique of "the original infantile story"

In *Madness and Modernism*, Louis Sass (2017) utilizes phenomenological insights to question several long-standing explanatory traditions within psychoanalysis. He is critical of "psychoanalytic notions about the dominance of primitive instinctual forces," "primary-process" thinking, and [ideas of] self-world fusion [as] akin to infancy" (p. xxx). Sass is particularly critical of the unquestioning psychoanalytic reliance on "the regression-fixation model" (p. 316). Here it benefits us to cite Sass at length:

> In 1911, Sigmund Freud described schizophrenia as a profound regression to the most primitive stage of "infantile eroticism." Since then, nearly all psychoanalytic writers have interpreted this type of psychosis as involving a deep regression to "the original infantile story." They see the structures of schizophrenic consciousness as a return to an archaic mode of experience dominated by illogical primary-process thinking; by hallucinatory wish-fulfillment fantasy and raw, untamed instinct; by a state of primal fusion with the world; and by an absence or severe attenuation of "observing ego" (the capacity for self-conscious reflection and ironic distance from experience) . . . . The regression or fixation in question has sometimes been understood largely as a deficiency, resulting from defects of the ego, at other times more as a defense, a way of escaping anxieties that a more mature consciousness would be forced to recognize . . . [S]chizophrenic consciousness

[it is thought] involves lower stages of psychological existence characterized by . . . deterioration in conceptual powers . . . derangement of purposeful attention . . . little capacity to reflect on the self and on immediate experience . . . an inability to distinguish self from environment; and by a dominance of . . . primitive processes of merging with an object.

(2017, p. 6)

Such ideas are not limited to psychoanalysis. A great many psychiatrists and psychologists since Freud's time have been influenced by this way of thinking, viewing schizophrenic disorder, for example, as a "lowering of the mental level," a "primary insufficiency of mental activity," or a reduction of psychic operations, and as "human activity in its simplest and most rudimentary forms" (Sass, 2017, p. 5). Sass is right, of course, to note that such formulations have a mechanistic cast, and that schizophrenic consciousness has accordingly been conceived as a malfunctioning computer that has been subject "to various kinds of 'defect,' 'deficit,' or 'failure' . . . such as impairment . . . defective capacity . . . or diminished ability" (2017, p. 5). What such conceptualizations typically sideline is the idea – championed by Sass – that there is a superabundance of cognitive functioning in schizophrenia and that the psychotic subject might play an active role in their delusions. Similarly sidelined – turning more directly to the Lacanian perspective that will be advanced here – is the idea that such delusions can be understood as creative attempts at recovery, as a part of what Leader (2016) has referred to as the *work* of psychosis.

To clarify, the argument I seek to make here is not that psychoanalytic thinkers have intentionally wielded a derogatory set of concepts in thinking about psychosis. There is considerable evidence to suggest that psychoanalytic thinking represented a significant humane advance on the earlier historical understandings and treatment practices regards madness/psychosis (Porter, 2003; Scull, 2015). I appreciate that the previously used terminology emerged from a psychoanalytic meta-psychology in which developmental conceptualizations played a foundational part. I acknowledge also that such ideas were the result of clinical theorizing within the sphere of psychopathology and that they can be said to retain clinical value. I note, moreover, that these conceptualizations were motivated by curative as opposing to devaluing agendas. All this being said, it is hard to deny the omnipresence of implicitly derogating language in these psychoanalytic conceptualizations ("primitive," "infantile," "illogical," "untamed," "defects," "deterioration," "derangement," "little capacity") which Sass (2017) has brought to our attention. Although Sass does not mention it specifically, references to narcissism (either in relation to psychosis or apart from it) likewise entail devaluing (if not downright pejorative) language, as Heinz Kohut (1966), a key theorist in the field, has warned. Narcissism is all too easily viewed as inferior, Kohut notes, as a state of self-love that is "more primitive" and "less adaptive" (1966, p. 61) than object love.

Importantly, I do not think that these conceptualizations account for all that psychoanalysis has or can say about psychosis, or for that matter, narcissism – hence our turn to Lacanian theory. Interestingly, despite the critique previously cited, Sass notes that "[the approach of] . . . the psychoanalyst Jacques Lacan may be an exception [to such explanatory trends in psychoanalysis]" (2017, p. xxx).[1] One of my objectives in this chapter is to show exactly why I believe that Sass's intuition regards Lacan's work is indeed correct.

John Nash: scenes from life

John Nash's autobiographical essay begins with a curiously phrased statement: "My beginning as a legally recognized individual occurred on June 13, 1928 in Bluefield, West Virginia" (Nash, 1994/2002, p. 5). While no doubt true, this assertion implies that for Nash, there may have been another existence outside or, or beyond, that as a "legally recognized individual." Nash continues: "My father, for whom I was named, was an electrical engineer" (1994/2002, p. 5), adding that this was a career he himself had considered prior to entering Carnegie Tech. Nash's mother, Margaret Virginia, had graduated from the University of West Virginia, and was an English school teacher prior to marrying Nash's father.

Nash, it appears, was a largely solitary child who devoted much of his spare time to reading and science experiments. It was suggested that he was a mathematical prodigy and he remembers being called "bug-brains" because of his "buggy ideas" (Nash, cited in Samels, 2002). In high school, Nash read "the classic 'Men of Mathematics' by E.T. Bell," which resulted in his experimenting with and ultimately "succeeding in proving the classic Fermat theorem about an integer multiplied by itself" (Nash, 1994/2002, p. 6), a notable accomplishment for a high schooler.

Nash won a Westinghouse Scholarship to fund his studies at Carnegie Tech. The supplementary math course that Nash took during his last year of schooling in Bluefield stood him in good stead: "I had advanced knowledge and ability and didn't need to learn much from the first math courses at Carnegie" (Nash, 1994/2002, p. 7). Rather than following accepted models or instructions for how to solve mathematical problems, Nash proved fiercely independent:

No one was more obsessed with originality . . . [or] more disdainful of authority . . . he was surrounded by the high priests of twentieth-century science – Albert Einstein, John von Neumann, and Norbert Weiner – but he joined no school, became no one's discipline. . . . In almost everything he did – from game theory to geometry – he thumbed his nose at the received wisdom. . . . Nash acquired his knowledge of mathematics not mainly from studying what other mathematicians discovered, but by rediscovering their truths for himself

(Nasar, 1998, p. 12).

Nash reputedly received a one-sentence recommendation from the Carnegie Institute when he graduated: "This man is a genius" (Samels, 2002). While Nash was offered fellowships by both Harvard and Princeton, the Princeton fellowship was, he felt, more generous, particularly given that "I had not actually won the Putnam competition" (1994/2002, p. 7). Nash's choice of words seems telling. His phrasing ("I had not actually won") suggests – and this is borne out by Nasar (1998) – that the highly prestigious mathematics award was something that he had become preoccupied with.

Despite being interested in all areas of mathematics – particular those in which he might be able to make a big splash (Samels, 2002) – Nash remained interested in the ideas in economics that he had been exposed to at Carnegie. This led to an interest in game theory and the work of John von Neumann, who was a professor at Princeton during Nash's time there. Von Neumann had had the idea that social behavior could be analyzed as two-person, zero-sum games. Nash's subsequent breakthrough was to shift Von Neumann's focus from the group to the individual, to move from zero-sum games to situations in which there was a mix of cooperative and noncooperative elements and in which, crucially, there was a possibility of mutual gain. Nash's resulting theory, subsequently to be known as "the Nash Equilibrium," would be the basis of his elegant 27-page doctoral dissertation.

While Nash had hoped to receive a faculty position at Princeton, this did not materialize. He eventually accepted a position at the Massachusetts Institute of Technology (MIT), which, significantly, he considered a second-rate institution – a fact underlined by its physical proximity to Harvard. Up until this point, Nash's mathematics career had been on a constantly upward trajectory. As Nasar puts it: "Nash's insights and discoveries had won him recognition, respect . . . He had carved out a brilliant career . . . become famous" (1998, p. 15). The relative comedown (at least in his own eyes) of an MIT appointment and a beckoning suburban existence with his pregnant wife Alicia, seemed to represent the end of this upward ascent. Added to this was a disappointment that Nash reports in his autobiographical essay:

> I studied . . . [a] problem involving partial differential equations which I had learned of as a problem that was unsolved . . . although I did succeed in solving the problem . . . it happened that I was working in parallel with Ennio de Giorgi [who] . . . was first actually to achieve the ascent of the summit . . . [if] de Giorgi . . . had failed in the attack on this problem . . . then the lone climber reaching the peak would have been recognized with mathematics' Fields medal.
>
> (1994/2002, p. 9)

The Fields Medal, even more that the Putnam competition, clearly represented an important ideal for Nash, something that had become central to his identity.

At around this time (late 1957), as Capps (2011) describes, Nash's increasingly erratic and irrational behavior was being noticed by his colleagues at MIT:

> This behavior included his appearance at a New Year's Eve costume party dressed only in diapers . . . announcing that he was the 1958 New Year's Eve Baby and spending the better part of the evening curled up in Alicia's lap, a performance that some partygoers found bizarre . . . his belief that his photograph on the cover of *Life* magazine had been disguised to make it look as if [he] were Pope John the 23rd; his complaints that his career was being ruined by aliens from outer space; his belief that his room at home was "bugged"; his letters addressed to foreign ambassadors, the UN, the Pope, and the F.B.I. that intimated that he was seeking to form a world government; his insistence on driving to Washington, D.C. to deliver the letters personally; his suspicion that a colleague was rifling through his waste basket in order to steal his ideas; his observation of men in red ties around the MIT campus who in his head had some relation to a crypto-communist party; his disorganized lecture at the American Mathematical Society meeting in which the math, according to a friend, "was just lunacy"; and his rejection of a prestigious chair at the University of Chicago on the grounds that he was soon to become the emperor of Antarctica.
>
> (p. 147)

What followed was a decade of psychotic suffering:

> For the next three decades, Nash suffered from severe delusions, hallucinations, disordered thought and feeling, and a broken will . . . [he] abandoned mathematics, embraced numerology and religious prophecy, and believed himself to be a "messianic figure of great but secret importance." He fled to Europe several times, was hospitalized involuntarily half a dozen times for periods up to year and a half, was subject to all sorts of drug and shock treatments, experienced brief remissions and episodes of hope that lasted only a few months, and finally became a sad phantom who haunted Princeton University campus where he had once been a brilliant graduate student, oddly dressed, muttering to himself, writing mysterious messages on blackboards, year after year.
>
> (Nasar, 1998, pp. 16–17)

The periods of hospitalization that punctuated these decades – deeply resented by Nash – were often followed by periods of apparent stabilization and lucidity. As Nash put it: "[W]hen I had been long enough hospitalized I would finally renounce my delusional hypotheses and revert to thinking of myself as a human of more conventional circumstance and return to mathematical research" (1994/2002,

p. 10). The intensity of psychotic delusions quietened as the 1970s arrived, when, as Nash reflects:

> I became a person of delusionally influenced thinking but of relatively moderate behavior and thus avoid hospitalization. . . . Gradually I began to intellectually reject some of the delusionally influenced lines of thinking which had been characteristic of my orientation. This began, most recognizably, with the rejection of politically-oriented thinking as essentially a hopeless waste of intellectual effort.
>
> (1994/2002, p. 10)

And yet, while Nash could say in 1994 that "at the present time I seem to be thinking rationally again in the style . . . of scientists," he added that this was "not entirely a matter of joy as if someone returned from physical disability to good health" because "rationality of thought imposes a limit on a person's concept of his relation to the cosmos" (1994/2002, p. 10).

While it is difficult to ascribe Nash's stabilization to any factor, both Nasar (1998) and Nash's wife Alicia felt that his being allowed to return to Princeton – albeit in an informal capacity, roaming the halls, writing on blackboards – was of considerable importance. One might also speculate that receiving the Nobel Memorial Prize in Economic Sciences in 1994, despite potentially being a disruptive or stressful event, perhaps played its part in helping to anchor Nash's identity as precisely the genius mathematician that he seemed so keen – so seemingly arrogantly – to perform in his younger years.

Refuting the diagnosis of Nash as a "highly narcissistic personality"

In the course of a series of articles on John Nash, Donald Capps (2003, 2004a, 2004b, 2005) draws on a variety of psychoanalytic ideas – including those of Freud, Erik Erikson, and Heinz Kohut – to advance a psychoanalytic conceptualization of Nash's psychotic breakdown. A central contention in these papers is that Nash had a narcissistic personality structure, and that as a result, as Capps states, "the psychological process that undergirded Nash's grandiose delusions was narcissism" (2004b, p. 294). My critique of Capps will focus on this contention. I will argue that such a conceptualization proves not only inadequate but also, ultimately, clinically misleading. It is important to provide a brief overview of Capps's argument as to why Nash was best categorized as possessing a narcissistic personality structure. As part of this overview, it will become apparent that there are facets of Capps's argument that I agree with, even though how I go on to articulate these points of agreement leads to a very different clinical presentation of the material.

How then does Capps apply the idea of narcissistic personality structure to Nash? He begins by drawing attention to one of the most pronounced features of the early stages of Nash's psychotic breakdown: the apparent megalomania evinced in Nash's grandiose delusions. Evidence of this sort is not hard to come by. Capps notes the importance of Nash's interest in the prophet Zarathustra, stressing that Nash felt "he was a figure akin to Zarathustra" (p. 294). He goes on to cite Nasar's (1998) comment that during his most delusional period, Nash believed that he was "a Messianic godlike figure with secret ideas" (Nasar, 1998, p. 335). Capps then appeals to Freud's (1911) study of Judge Daniel Paul Schreber so as to substantiate the claim that "megalomania or highly grandiose beliefs about one-self have a basis in paranoia" (p. 294), adding also that "paranoid delusions may be traced to . . . a fixation in sexual development around the psychodynamics of narcissism" (p. 294). If one accepts the idea that megalomania might have a basis in paranoia – and I am not necessarily in disagreement with Capps on this point – it raises an obvious objection: surely what undergirds Nash's psychology is less narcissism than paranoia? This is a point I will return to. For Capps, presumably, a fixation in sexual development of a narcissistic sort is, by contrast, the crucial factor, although, as he himself concedes, this remains necessarily speculative given the lack of any real substantiating evidence. Capps is, however, quick to qualify that "What is not speculative . . . is [Nash's] . . . narcissism" (p. 294).

What follows is a rather strained attempt to justify this diagnosis. Capps begins with the claim that "Nash took particular pride in his body" (p. 297), citing by way of corroboration the remarks of several of Nash's peers as reported by Naser (Nash was, for example, thought to have had "a very strong, very muscular body," to be as "handsome as a god," to have "the look of an English Aristocrat" [Naser, 1998, p. 67]). This is troublesome. Although there may be good evidence that Nash possessed a desirable physique and that many of his peers found him highly attractive, none of this has any direct bearing on whether or not Nash was narcis-sistically structured. This much would seem obvious: attributions made of Nash's physical features cannot be the basis of diagnostic speculation. Capps's argument is at its weakest here.

A second apparent diagnostic indicator that Capps calls upon concerns the idea of the "defense against affects" (p. 298) which he takes to be characteristic of narcissism. Capps sees the related phenomenon of "withdrawal of feeling from [the] . . . body" (p. 298) as exemplified in Nash's response to the death of his childhood playmate Herman Kirchner and in his later response to the death of his father. This defense is then linked to Naser's comments on "Nash's inability to imagine how his actions affected other people" (1998, p. 209). Problems arise here as well. Such a "defense against affects" is a less than definitive criterion for narcissism given that it may be just as – if not *more* – easily associated with obsessional neurosis. It is as such a poor criterion for any attempt at a differential diagnosis. One should note also that there is something of a disjunction in Capps's argument: a defense against one's own affects is not necessarily the same as a cognitive inability to imagine how one's actions might affect others.

A third theme of diagnostic importance for Capps involves Nash's commit-ment to achieving the highest possible level of recognition within mathematics.

In the intellectual hierarchy of MIT, says Capps, paraphrasing the comments of several of Nash's fellow students, "mathematics was the highest thing" and "Nash was the closest thing to royalty" (cited in Nasar, 1998, p. 196). One of Nash's peers commented that "He wanted to be noticed more than anything" (Nasar, p. 67), a view affirmed by Nasar herself: "he seized opportunities to boast about his accomplishments" (p. 67). Without in any way doubting the truth of such claims, we might nevertheless ask: an ambitious craving for recognition is not, surely, the sole preserve of narcissists? Once again, this seems a less than definitive criterion for a diagnosis of narcissistic structure. In fairness, however, Capps adds a further dynamic consideration here by emphasizing that Nash's "grandiose self image . . . was thoroughly shattered by [a] . . . humiliating experience" (p. 302). He has in mind Nash's catastrophic performance at the American Mathematical Society in 1959 where he presented – in a barely coherent and a largely nonsensical manner – his theory on the Riemann Hypothesis, one of the most vexing problems in the history of mathematics. Capps once again cites Freud's (1911) study of Schreber to argue that a frequent cause of paranoia involves a severe injury to the ego and its ideals. I think Capps is right to highlight the importance of this event in Nash's breakdown. His use of Freud is, however, misleading; Freud is primarily concerned with paranoia rather than narcissism in the context of the Schreber case. Once again, we are confronted with the question as to why narcissism and not paranoia is given a structural role in the conceptualization of Nash's psychosis.

Capps seems in a muddle here over whether paranoia or narcissism plays the predominant role. To recap, there is, on the one hand, the view that narcissism is itself founded upon paranoia. As Capps himself puts it: "megalomania or highly grandiose beliefs about the self have a basis in paranoia. This was certainly true in Nash's case" (p. 294). And yet, on the other hand, and as we have seen, Capps also wants to suggest that "a fixation in . . . the psychodynamics of narcissism" (p. 294) is of foundational importance when it comes to paranoid delusions. Upon reflection, the first of these two arguments proves more compelling, for the simple reason that the second seems circular: it presumes what it claims to explain. Recall that for Capps, megalomania and grandiosity are seen as arising from paranoia, which itself is the outcome of a narcissistic fixation. This is dangerously close to being tautologous: narcissism (as libidinal fixation) is being used to account for grandiosity and megalomania (that is, narcissism in its more extreme forms). That narcissism causes grandiosity seems, after all, a less than effective explanation if narcissism and grandiosity are effectively synonyms. Where such a style of explanation fails is that it does not investigate thoroughly enough what really motivates and underlies the grandiosity in question. Differently put: what if the grandiosity in question is something more than an echo of the presumed diagnosis of narcissistic personality structure? We need thus to dig a little deeper, to see what underlies these narcissistic features.

One might raise an objection at this point. There is, surely, a crucial difference between a residual degree of healthy narcissism and the more exaggerated or psychotic forms of megalomania and grandiosity as evinced by Nash. This much, I concede. Nonetheless, my problematization of Capps's clinical reasoning remains relevant at least in so far as it encourages us not to simply accept the all-too-readily available "explanation" of narcissism. It prompts us to enquire what underlies narcissistic symptomology other than narcissism itself. From a Lacanian standpoint, the megalomania and delusions of grandiosity that Capps so emphasizes within Nash's biography should not be viewed simply as the outcome of a narcissistic personality structure. Rather – and here I anticipate the argument I will develop in the coming pages – they might be seen as the result of a need stemming from an altogether different psychical structure, a need to substantiate and give definition to an inchoate and fundamentally imperiled sense of self.

One might argue that although there may have been evident shortcomings in the diagnostic evidence advanced by Capps, this does not mean that the overarching diagnosis that he suggested is necessarily inaccurate. True enough. There is indeed abundant evidence in biographical accounts of Nash's life that he acted in a narcissistic manner both prior to and during the onset of his psychotic decompensation. The crucial question, however, is whether we should view this evidence of narcissism as symptomatic or fundamentally structural in nature. In order to do this, it will help to highlight features of narcissism as foregrounded by two routinely cited authors in the domain of psychoanalytic psychopathology, namely Glen Gabbard (2014) and Nancy McWilliams (2011).

Before turning to the recent overview accounts of narcissism, it is worth briefly noting that to speak of narcissism, certainly within the colloquial terms of everyday speech, is to imply a value judgment. To speak then of someone as *structurally* narcissistic seems likewise to imply a pejorative moral evaluation, although at a more substantive level, even permitting that diagnostically, no such negatively inflected evaluation is necessarily intended. In the more technical terms of psychoanalytic conceptualization, to speak of narcissism is to imply a fragile yet relatively stable ego which requires constant reassurance of its own value (indeed, typically, of its own imagined superiority). McWilliams notes that: "The term 'narcissistic' refers to people whose personalities are organized around maintaining their self-esteem by getting affirmations from outside themselves" (2011, p. 176). McWilliams credits C.G. Jung with being the first analytic writer to describe the features of the grandiose narcissistic person, features including "exhibitionism, aloofness, emotional inaccessibility, fantasies of omnipotence, [the] overvaluation of [their own] creativity, and a tendency to be judgmental" (p. 178). Gabbard (2014) likewise identifies as narcissistic the features of "the arrogant, boastful, 'noisy' individual who demands to be in the spotlight . . . and clearly need[s] to be the center of attention" (p. 484). Narcissism, approached in these terms, involves more than excessive egotism; it entails also an economy of libidinal gratification, which is to say that the narcissistic not only craves but also *enjoys* (in Lacanian terms, "gets off on") the attention of others.

Both Gabbard (2014) and McWilliams (2011) highlight that there are two contrasting modalities of narcissism. In the psychoanalytic literature, notes

Gabbard, there is a continuum stretching from "the envious, greedy individual who demands attention and acclaim of others" (the type of narcissism described by Otto Kernberg), to a type of narcissistic personality that is "more vulnerable to slights and self fragmentation" (as studied by Heinz Kohut) (Gabbard, 2014, p. 484).[2] This distinction is often understood as the difference between *oblivious* and *hypervigilant* types or narcissism, as a contrast between "exhibitionistic" and "closet" or between "thick-skinned" and "thin-skinned" types (McWilliams, 2011). This being said, it is nonetheless the case for McWilliams that narcissistic people of all appearances share "an inner sense of, and/or terror of insufficiency, shame, weakness . . . inferiority [and] . . . a narcissistic hunger for recognition" (p. 179). Criteria for narcissistic personality disorder as listed in the *DSM-5* (American Psychiatric Association, 2013) accordingly include the following features: a grandiose sense of self-importance, a preoccupation with fantasies of unlimited success, a need for excessive admiration, a deficit of empathic ability, unwillingness to recognize the feelings of others, and haughty behaviors or attitudes.

Interestingly, both Gabbard and McWilliams offer cautionary notes in respect to diagnoses of narcissism. "Narcissistic personality organization seems currently over-diagnosed," says McWilliams (2011), adding that: "The concept is often misapplied to people having situation specific reactions" or to those with "depressive, obsessive compulsive, and hysterical personalities" (p. 192). Gabbard (2014) warns that the concept "is almost always used pejoratively, especially when referring to . . . [those] whom we find unpleasant," stressing also that "it is often problematic to determine which traits indicate a narcissistic personality . . . and which are simply adaptive" (p. 482).

So, are we able to identify any of these stated symptoms of narcissism in Nash's biography? Well, according to Nasar (1998), Nash seemed always to put his own interests first, paying little heed to the needs and feelings of others:

> All through his childhood, adolescence, and brilliant career, Nash seemed . . . immune to the emotional forces that bind people together . . . while he was preoccupied with the effects of others on him, he mostly ignored – indeed, seemed unable to grasp – his effect on others. . . . He wished the others to be satisfied by his genius"
>
> (Nasar, 1998, pp. 167–168).

Nasar, despite being a conscientiously even-handed biographer, goes on to comment that Nash "behaved selfishly, even callously" (p. 179) in making the "cold-blooded suggestion" (p. 178) that his first son, John David, be given up for adoption despite the protestations of the boy's mother, Eleanor Stier. Eleanor – whom Nash refused to marry – believed that Nash "gave no sign that he understood, even remotely, what such a separation might mean for a mother or her child" (p. 176).

Evidence of this sort is not hard to come by. Nonetheless, for reasons that will soon become clear, I maintain that Nash's narcissistic behaviors need not be considered properly *structural* in nature. To make such an assumption, to leap from symptomatic behaviors to a conclusion about underlying psychic structure, is, certainly within the terms of Lacanian psychoanalysis, to risk a fundamental diagnostic error. (I might note here, parenthetically, that such an error seems omnipresent – indeed, virtually impossible to avoid – in our current *DSM-5* era of symptom-based diagnoses). This apparent error is compounded by another. From a Lacanian standpoint, the concept of narcissism cannot be utilized or understood in a structural capacity. Why not? Well, for Lacan, any of the basic structures of subjectivity (that is, neurosis, psychosis and perversion) can exhibit narcissistic traits or behaviors without narcissism being the overall organizing or structural factor. Narcissism, moreover, is considered inadequate as a deciding factor in any differential diagnosis precisely because it is an inherent aspect of *any* ego. (One is reminded of Freud (1914) in this respect: "narcissism . . . [is] the libidinal complement to the egoism of the instinct of self-preservation, a measure of which may justifiably be attributed to every living creature" [pp. 73–74].) If this Lacanian claim holds water – and it helps here to hear out the argument – then to elevate narcissism to the status of a structural concept risks confusion at a more foundational level, obscuring more elementary diagnostic considerations, such as asking whether a given subject is structurally psychotic or neurotic. The accounts advanced by Capps (2003, 2004a, 2004b, 2005) suffer, I think, from just such diagnostic confusions.

Evidence of narcissistic behavior, is, for Lacanians, not the end of a diagnostic debate. Such evidence prompts instead the questions: "Narcissistic how?"; "Narcissistic to what ends?"; and "Narcissistic in terms of what broader libidinal economy?" Approached with these questions in mind, it becomes clear that Nash's narcissistic actions and behaviors are of a very particular sort. They seem less an instance of a gratuitous "libidinal investment of the self" (to use Kohut's [1966, p. 243] descriptive phrase) and more of an ego survival strategy. At the beginning of this section, I listed a series of characterizing features of narcissism, including the ideas that narcissistic personalities lack self-esteem, crave the recognition of others, possess an inner sense of insufficiency, maintain a grandiose sense of self-importance, etc., etc. I suggested also – my own description, admittedly – that the narcissist subject, following the accounts of Gabbard (2014) and McWilliams (2011), could be described as having a fragile yet basically stable ego. What, though, if such characterizations, especially once applied to someone like Nash, presume too much? All of the previously stated portrayals presume a basically viable ego. What, though, if the basic operational assumption of an "I" – in Lacanian terms, the self-substantializing function of the ego – turns out to be less than secure?

If we are dealing with a subject for whom an overarching ego structure cannot be assumed, for whom the very question of personal identity represents a fundamental impasse, their ostensibly narcissistic actions presumably play a role that goes beyond mere egotism or libidinal gratification. The role of narcissistic behavior under such circumstances is about something more rudimentary than a craving for the affirmation from others or the need to nurse an impoverished sense of self-esteem. Taking such a Lacanian possibility into account – the prospect, in other words, that Nash was psychotically structured prior to the actual trigger-ing of his most explicitly schizophrenic behaviors and delusions – dramatically changes how we view the features of the case. The pejorative value judgments that Gabbard (2014) warns against, which begin automatically to accrue when characterizations of narcissism are offered, are mitigated – if not altogether sus-pended – when we have a broader psychic context that helps to explain the func-tion of such behaviors. If a tentative diagnosis of psychotic structure – initially latent, and yet increasingly overt as the period of triggering approaches – holds in Nash's case, then, following Lacanian theory, we would need to foreground exactly the dilemma of ego-viability. We would need to stress the imperative, for a psychotically structured subject, of attaining a coherent, ongoing, and stable sense of personal identity. This dilemma is more rudimentary, more primary to the psy-chical suffering of the psychotic subject than are their ostensibly "psychopatho-logical" narcissistic features. It now becomes clear that precisely those features are not in and of themselves "pathological" at all; they are rather the subject's attempts at forestalling dissolution, at holding together an otherwise fragmentary set of subjective experiences. It is this level of suffering that needs to be fore-grounded in a prospective treatment.

It helps here to turn again to Nash's biography. A careful reading of Nasar's account of Nash's life suggests that his narcissistic behaviors were, in retrospect, not that of a particularly robust or adaptive ego. Many of Nash's behaviors and life choices were, I think, driven less by the libidinal gains of narcissism or by a perennial crisis of lacking self-esteem, than by a far more rudimentary need: that of attaining an elementary form of selfhood. This is the difference between a basically functional (if easily wounded) ego that is hungry for ego-gratification (the "loud narcissist" as described by Gabbard [2014]) and the desperate need of a psychotically structured subject to attain a rudimentary degree of ego-viability. A schematic distinction might prove helpful here. We might expect of a neurotic subject with narcissistic features (particularly of "exhibitionistic" type) that they would be hungry to have an idealized, grandiose self-image seen by others. (Don-ald Trump's tweeting of an image of his face on the muscular body of Sylvester Stallone's Rocky Balboa in November 2019 seems a perfect example). The psy-chotic subject evincing narcissistic behavior, by contrast, could be said to do so as a means of enacting the elementary ego-coherence that the neurotic takes for granted. Their goal is not, most fundamentally, the adulation of others; it is rather an attempt at consolidating a fragmenting ego.

If Nash was neurotically narcissistic, so we could argue, then a psychotic break-down would have been unlikely. It would have been unlikely for the reason that

Nash would have had the ability to summon up other anchoring images of himself, even in circumstances of severe subjective crisis. This neurotic resource – of being equipped with an imaginary supply of mirror-images of the self – would have kept him sane. Suffice to say, this was not a resource that Nash appeared to possess. For Nash, there was one image that needed continual upkeep and maintenance, that of the brilliant young upwardly mobile "genius" mathematician and future Fields Medal winner. When this image could not be sustained, then the first signs of psychotic decompensation became evident. If Nash was neurotically narcissistic, we should expect to see numerous examples of narcissistic wounding in his biography, perhaps alongside examples of rage at being affronted. What we find, by contrast, once we immerse ourselves in the biographical data, is not an abundance of evidence of narcissistic wounding but rather, when confronted with ego-threatening loss – such as being suddenly fired from the RAND Corporation, or the unexpected death of his namesake father – Nash responded not in a self-important or attention-demanding way, but in a muted fashion, with apparent confusion, as if he hadn't fully grasped what had occurred.[3] His response was one of withdrawal, of "remarkable detachment" as Nasar (1998, p. 187) puts it. Instead of the clamorous reactions of an all-important ego, one has here instead the impression of an ego being erased, of Nash's subjectivity fading into incoherence.

A very different perspective on Nash's ostensibly narcissistic personality now comes into view. Consider, for example, the remark by one of Nash's fellow students cited by Nasar (1998): "He wanted to be noticed more than anything" (p. 67), or the series of ostensibly egotistical character traits noted by Nasar (1998) herself: Nash boasting about his accomplishments, his apparent need for admiration, the fact that he would "consistently underscore his own uniqueness" (p. 145). Also worth reflecting upon is the remark Nash made to a colleague soon after he joined MIT: "[T]here are few geniuses these days at MIT. Me, of course, and also Norbert Weiner" (Nasar, p. 146). Telling also is Nasar's proclamation that "Nash craved a more universal form of recognition . . . based on what he regarded as an objective standard, uncolored by emotion or personal ties" (p. 44).

At first glance, these anecdotes seem instances of blatant narcissism – particularly perhaps Nash's proclaiming himself a genius – unless of course, we consider that the incessantly repeated image in question, that of the young mathematical genius, might have been what, to all intents and purposes, was keeping him sane. Reconsidering these anecdotes in light of the prospect that Nash was psychotically structured enables us to bring an altogether different clinical sensibility to the material. If, for example, one has a less than secure sense of one's own singular existence – a not uncommon experience for psychotic people – then what could be more important than having this precarious existence noticed, remarked upon, afforded a unique position? If, furthermore, Nash was reliant upon a particular image of himself as a means of maintaining a minimal degree of ego-coherence, then we should not be surprised if he often affirmed that image (of a mathematical genius) to others, or, as seems likely in the preceding example, he sought to consolidate it via reference to the image of like others (other figures of genius) to which he compared himself. Continuing this line of speculation: Nasar's insightful comment that Nash preferred an *objective* rather than a merely subjective form of recognition suggests that Nash was ultimately less interested in the adulation of others (precisely what the textbook narcissist yearns for) and more intent on securing a permanent symbolic marker that might consolidate an otherwise precarious sense of singular existence and subjective coherence.

John Nash's work of psychosis

In the opening pages of this chapter, I suggested that for Lacanians, one can speak meaningfully of the work of psychosis. This idea is essentially an extension of Freud's (1914) postulate that various symptoms of psychosis can be understood as attempts at recovery. Speaking of the Scherber case, Freud remarked: "What we take to be the pathological production, the delusional formation, is in reality the attempt at recovery, the reconstruction" (Freud, 1911, p. 71). Interestingly, Capps (2004b, 2005) notes this idea repeatedly (reminding readers of "Freud's view that delusions are an attempt at recovery" [2004b, p. 290]), but seems not to register its deeper significance for his own argument. If we take seriously the idea that delusions represent an attempt at recovery, then it makes good clinical sense to ask what exactly the delusions are trying to achieve. If we take this approach – one which stresses the agency and creativity of the psychotic subject rather than focusing on the apparently maladaptive, dysfunctional, or regressive nature of their delusions – then delusions should be viewed as agentic in nature, as a means of responding to often severe and seemingly insurmountable psychical difficulties. To take up this issue in more pragmatic clinical terms: delusions should be read as holding vital clues for the direction of the clinical work and how it might best facilitate stabilization.

In respect of Nash then, as argued previously, his grandiose delusions should be seen not simply as the ideational and behavioral echoes of a narcissistic structure. They can instead be read as attempts at attaining that which he was most lacking and seemingly desperate for: a position of singularity, a unique identity, or, differently put, something akin to a viable, adaptive ego that would substantiate and give definition to an inchoate and imperiled sense of self. If this is true, then the diagnosis of a narcissistic ego has it completely wrong. Nash's psychosis was not the enactment of narcissism, not the outcome of an ego craving self-esteem or the ego-gratifying attentions of others; it was more the survival strategy of a subject who appeared to lack a viable ego (or "I-function") apart from the image of the young, brilliant mathematical genius. The grandiosity of Nash's delusions appears now in a different light.

The very hyperbolic nature of Nash's delusory identifications (as Emperor of Antarctica, as Messianic god-like figure) can be read as overcompensatory attempts to attain the sense of subjective singularity that he so desperately lacked.

Picking highly distinct – if overtly fictitious – historical personages, seems, given this psychical context, a perfect (even if unconscious) strategy. After all, what better way to secure a sense of a distinctive and valued existence than to assume the identity of a figure who has occupied a unique position in the history of humankind? As gratuitously over the top as an identification as the Emperor of Antarctica might be, you are unlikely ever to forget him, or indeed, mistake him for anyone else, once you have met him. It is interesting in this respect that Nash's winning of the Nobel Prize in 1994 correlated with a sustained period of stabilization. While a series of other factors no doubt played their part here, one could speculate that winning the Nobel finally afforded Nash the objective symbolic recognition that he had so badly needed (recall Nasar's [1998] remark that "Nash craved a more universal form of recognition . . . based on what he regarded as an objective standard, uncolored by emotion or personal ties" [p. 44]). The Nobel Prize arguably secured for him a singular historical position, providing the necessary symbolic supports for him to consolidate what had all but ceased to function during his psychotic breakdown – a viable ego.

Once again, the shortcomings of viewing Nash as narcissistically structured becomes apparent. Speaking of Nash's fascination with the figure of Zarathustra, Capps (1994b) notes "Zarathustra became the prophetic leader of millions . . . and gained a lasting place in the annals of human history" (p. 294). Capps subsequently takes up Nash's preoccupation with Zarathustra as evidence of his (Nash's) narcissism, rather than explore what really necessitated such fascinations and prospective identifications in the first place. Capps thus fails thus to grasp that it may have been the absolute singularity of Zarathustra's historical identity that motivated Nash's interest in him, rather than Nash's own prospective grandiosity. Capps seems also to miss the stabilizing value that winning the Nobel Prize appeared to have for Nash, commenting that whereas "Zarathustra became . . . [a] prophetic leader . . . Nash [needed to] be content with a Nobel Prize in economics. A great honor . . . but not in the same league with the immortal Zarathustra" (p. 294).

There is, at this late stage of the chapter, little room to add a further level of Lacanian theory to my reconceptualization of John Nash's psychosis. That being said, I would like to add one further note concerning how John Nash made creative recourse to the symbolic domain in his delusions, a type of recourse that was, I think, very much an attempt at recovery. It will be necessary, as part of such an account, to introduce a useful Lacanian idea, namely, that of *making an appeal to another register*. This is a key facet of Lacan's reading, in his fourth seminar, *The Object Relation* (2020), of Freud's case of Little Hans (Freud, 1909) who, famously, suffered from horse phobia. At the time of Freud's intervention, Hans found himself in a perplexing situation, confronting a series of significant life changes that proved difficult for him to process (instances of the "real" in Lacanian parlance). There had, for a start, been a shift in the structure and dynamics of his family; his baby sister had recently been born. Hans was, moreover, experiencing his first erections. This budding sense of sexuality was made no easier by a permissive mother who seemed unwilling to enforce any definitive sexual prohibitions. Similarly, Hans' father seemed, perhaps due to his reading of Freud's theories, notably reticent to assume the role of a castrating Oedipal father.

Hans, in Lacan's reading, lacked an instantiation of law and prohibition (in Lacanian terminology, the "Name-of-the-Father"). What Hans needed, in other words, was something akin to a paternal operator, some embodiment of the Law (or, in more Freudian terms, an agent of castration), that would enable him to reorganize his world and to specify the rules pertaining to the new roles and relationships that he now needed to take on. Little Hans was, in other words, burdened with the task of how to relocate himself in a changed world, and to do so without the restructuring effects of a resolved Oedipus complex. How, for example, should he situate himself relative to his mother, father, and sister now that his family configuration had so definitely changed? What new system of rules and prohibitions should now be applied? Who, furthermore, should be identified with, or feared, or desired? What is now prohibited? Lacan's answer to what Little Hans was evidently lacking – the necessary components to induce an Oedipal crisis – is that a particular signifier needed to be drawn out of the symbolic domain and exaggerated, heavily invested with libido, and thereby given organizational properties. Hence, the phobic reaction Hans exhibits to horses (or, more accurately, to the signifier "horse"). Within the remit of the horse phobia, Lacan argues, Hans finds something at once larger than life and fear inducing, something that enables him to reorder the co-ordinates of his puzzling family and symbolic situation.

What is crucial to Lacan is the idea that this paternal operator – the signifier "horse" – entails the type of flexibility and artificiality that only a signifier can provide. Indeed, the signifier "horse" represents multiple different shifting meanings and values for Hans across the duration of the case). As Leader (2011) explains:

> [With] the horse he [Hans] created a grammar that included all the aspects of his everyday life. The horse could bite or not bite, fall down or remain upright, be attached to carriages or not, and so on. Hans was creating a system to reorder his world, creating prohibitions as to what he could do or not do, where he could go or not go, through the phobic object – the horse – that he was using as his instrument . . . it was a way of appealing to the symbolic function of the father where the real father had let him down. It was the horse and not the father that became the mythical, frightening, powerful figure that was to literally reorder his world. The phobia was a properly creative process.
>
> (p. 54)

For Lacan then, it was precisely through an appeal to the symbolic dimension – the domain of signifiers, of laws, of the operations of language – that Hans was able to mediate and reorganize his world. It is vital to stress here that the symbolic is a *different register*: such a paternal operator ("horse") allowed Hans to reorganize the imaginary world of relations and familial roles precisely because it came *from outside* that imaginary domain. It was not merely one more imaginary object within his everyday world; it came an altogether different level of reality. This is, likewise, a crucial aspect of Lacan's theory of the Name-of-the-Father, which maintains that any instance of paternity needs something outside of itself – something, precisely, from another register, from the symbolic domain – to confer upon it the effects of authority and power that the role of Father comes to be invested with in patriarchal societies.[4] We begin to appreciate then how a privileged master signifier – such as, paradigmatically, the Name-of-the-Father – can be used a means of "treating the real," of modifying one's relationship to a series of imaginary intersubjective relations.

Lacan's idea of an appeal to another register perhaps helps explain the outlandish nature of Nash's claims at the time of his breakdown. The signifiers that he was drawing upon ("the Emperor of Antarctica," etc.) to try to reconfigure his troubling imaginary realm were precisely disproportionate in the sense previously described. They were extraordinary, "overly fictitious" (the very stuff of science fiction, in many instances). The very excessive quality which ensured that such signifiers seemed so crazy, so unbelievable to others, might have been precisely what made them serviceable for Nash. If he was to find an effectively disproportionate signifier, a signifier able to stand outside of – and indeed, to reorganize – the confusing and threatening elements of his imaginary environment, then such a signifier would clearly need to be selected from beyond the parameters of the ordinary.[5]

For those of us who are nonpsychotic, who already possess such a disproportionate signifier (the Name-of-the-Father), and who benefit from the structuring subjective effects that accrue to it, conventional social norms and meanings are firmly anchored. The same is true of the overarching parameters of symbolic identity; although such identities may be subject to much neurotic questioning and problematization, they remain stable and unlikely to be suddenly uprooted. Such processes have already occurred developmentally, and consistent self-experience and ego-coherence is the result. From such a perspective, anyone who attempts to self-initiate such a process, to independently select and elevate a signifier to a position akin to that of the Name-of-the-Father, is to appear erratic and eccentric at best, and at worst, pathological, mad.

I mention this so as to stress two points. First, while it understandable that the attempt to use a delusion to reorganize one's world (in Lacanian terms, this is referred to as the use of the "delusional metaphor") may appear to nonpsychotic people as odd, disturbed, crazy, etc., there is in fact nothing intrinsically pathological or dysfunctional about this process. There are, indeed, many structural parallels precisely with the function of Name-of-the-Father, which serves, after all, as the underpinning of everyday neurotic subjectivity. Second, while not inherently pathological, such attempts to instantiate an organizing master signifier (be it in the form of a temporary paternal operator or a delusional metaphor) require considerable symbolic labor and creativity. We need bear in mind also that such a process is happening precisely outside the parameters of conventionality (the operation of the Name-of-the-Father, by contrast, locates the neurotic subject firmly within the symbolic order, installing a compass of symbolic values and norms). It entails as such the ever-present prospect of social ostracization. Moreover, given that the use of such provisional organizing master signifiers seldom attains the structural fixity of the Name-of-the-Father, such attempts at stabilization are never over, but require constant – and often, taxing and exhausting – upkeep. All of this is to say that, rather than being viewed as dysfunctional, maladaptive, regressive etc., delusions – and this is characteristic of a Lacanian orientation to psychosis more generally (Leader, 2011, 2016; Rogers, 2016; Vanheule, 2011, 2020) – should be respected rather than pathologized.

Conclusion

Looking back on the analysis provided in this chapter, one might ask: how successful is a Lacanian approach in avoiding the derogations and devaluations that, following Sass (2017), invariably characterize standard psychoanalytic accounts of psychosis? We could follow that by asking: how successful is a Lacanian perspective in avoiding a deficit model conceptualization when it comes to psychosis?

In respect of the first question, I would argue that the Lacanian ideas advanced here do offer some modest steps toward a more emancipatory perspective on psychotic suffering. This seems the case particularly in respect to how the notion of narcissistic personality (and the pejorative values that have become typically associated with it) might be rethought in the context of psychotic structure. Behaviors such as Nash's that might otherwise have been attributed to narcissistic personality structure are, I think, given a more sympathetic hearing when viewed within the parameters of psychotic structure. The obvious retort to such a suggestion would simply be to note that psychotic structure – even once articulated in Lacanian terms that ideally imply no value judgment on what is a naturally occurring and often viable nonpathological psychic structure – nonetheless brings with it a series of devaluing connotations all of its own.[6] A firmer step toward an emancipatory stance on psychosis can be found in the Lacanian emphasis on delusions as modes of recovery and the associated notion of the delusional metaphor as a way of stabilizing triggered forms of psychosis (Lacan, 1993; Redmond, 2014; Vanheule, 2011, 2020; Ver Eecke, 2019). Regrettably, given limited space, we have not been able to explore these ideas in any real detail. They are, nonetheless, steps in the right direction when it comes to de-pathologizing psychotic symptoms and in encouraging a more emancipatory attitude in clinicians, who might come to respect and play the role of witness and student with regard to the delusional productions of patients.

In response to the second question, I refer to the work of my colleague Stijn Vanheule (2011). Speaking of Lacan's work of the 1950s, in which the idea of the foreclosure of the Name-of-the-Father remained the key explanatory concept in respect of psychosis, Vanheule remarks:

> No matter how strongly Lacan argued that psychosis should not be studied in terms of inherent defects . . . his concept of foreclosure still implied that compared to neurosis a signifier is lacking . . . [This] suggests that psychosis is marked by a fundamental flaw.
>
> (Vanheule, 2011, pp. 136–137)

Lacan's work in the 1960s understands psychosis very differently, along the lines of *an act of faith* (in the Other) *not having taken place*. Neurosis and psychosis are not considered to be paradigmatically different in terms of how the symbolic domain is composed, but rather in terms of how it is comes to be effectively used by the subject. This, for Vanheule (2011), implies a decisive shift away from a deficit model:

> [Lacan's] redefinition of the Name-of-the-Father in terms of an act of faith . . . enables us to break with a deficit model of psychosis. . . . The idea of [the installation or non-installation of] a belief in the Other as guarantee . . . does not focus on failure but diversity . . . [These are] are two positions for the . . . subject . . . Lacan [correspondingly] . . . takes a positive view on the a-subjective dimension in psychosis.
>
> (2011, p. 147)

In Lacan's work of the 1960s, psychosis and neurosis are seen "as just different 'subject structures,' different logics by means of which sense is made of the world . . . [i]n both structures normality is possible, just like in both the subject can suffer" (Vanheule, 2011, p. 137). While engaging with Vanheule's argument in detail is obviously not possible in the space that remains, it does lead us to pose a question in respect to Nash's psychosis as seen through a Lacanian lens. We know, in the terms of the Lacanian theory described in this chapter, that the psychotically structured subject lacks a firm anchoring in the symbolic order (the Name-of-the-Father not being operative). As such, they cannot rely on the symbolic conventions and norms that have been so thoroughly installed in neurotics. The psychotic subject is thus obliged to invent. Instead of relying on the framework of given symbolic meanings and consensual social narratives, they need to find their own way of articulating existing symbolic elements. This symbolic labor, as previously discussed, provides a way of anchoring meaning and grounding one's own identity and social relations. Is this not precisely what we see repeatedly in Nash's life, namely that his mathematical genius was predicated precisely on him needing to formulate problems – and solutions – in his own unique way? Could we say then that what effectively made John Nash a genius was the very fact of his psychotic structure? From a Lacanian perspective, the answer would be: yes.

Notes

1 This is perhaps unsurprising in view of Lacan's critical perspective on the notion of regression. The notion of regression seemed, to Lacan – at least in the hands of post-Freudian psychoanalysts – overly reliant on an initial assumption that the time of the psyche is, in its normative state, linear in nature (Evans, 1996). This is too much of an assumption for Lacan – and a broader Lacanian critique of the use of developmental thinking in psychoanalysis comes into view here (see Hook, 2017) – for a series of good Freudian reasons. For Lacan, we need to take seriously Freud's thoughts on the temporality of the unconscious (which does not abide by a linear or chronological partitioning of time), his insistence on the ongoing existence of the primary process (which has no sense of developmental progress), and his emphasis on the retroactivity of psychical life – Freud's notion of deferred action, or *nachtraglikheit*, being the crucial consideration here (Wang, 2019). If we foreground these notions, then we cannot, for Lacan, assume that the linear temporality implied by notions of development and regression alike should in fact be the default mode of temporality when it comes to the unconscious. This is not to say that Lacan completely avoids all mention of regression. Regression does, in fact, feature in his early accounts of psychosis. Importantly, however, this is what he calls topographical regression, regression to imaginary as opposed to symbolic modes of subjectivity (Lacan, 1993; Vanheule, 2011). One could argue, on the one hand, that such a conceptualization avoids to some extent the juvenilizing tendency present in chronologically oriented notions of regression. On the other hand, one would have to concede that even if regression is topographically conceptualized, it still does suggest a backward step of sorts, a more conflict-prone and an ultimately a less stable basis for subjectivity.

2 One objection to my critique of Capps could be mounted here. His account of Nash's narcissism is very much based on Kohut's model. As such, a rigorous critique of Capps should focus specifically on Kohut's ideas and avoid evoking more general conceptualizations of narcissism (such as those of Gabbard [2014] and McWilliams [2011]). While this is a valid comment, an extended critique of Capps via Kohut would require a far more detailed and analytically specific engagement than I am able to accommodate here. My overarching agenda in this chapter is to provide a Lacanian critique of how a concept like narcissism has been utilized by authors such as Capps in thinking about psychosis (hence, my introductory comments on the limitations of stylized forms of psychoanalytic explanation). Moreover, Capps himself does shift between theoreticians in his discussion of Nash, drawing on the work of Kernberg (1986) and Lowen (1983), among several others.

3 In respect to being unexpectedly fired from the RAND Corporation (where Nash was a consultant during his MIT years) for an act of sexual indecency, Nasar (1998) offers the following: "Nash did not appear shaken or embarrassed . . . Indeed, he seemed to be having trouble believing [the situation]. . . . He acted, weirdly, as if nothing had happened. He played the role of observer of his own drama . . . [he responded] with remarkable detachment" (Nasar, 1998, pp. 186–187). As regards the death of Nash's father, Nasar writes of Nash: "There was no outpouring of grief, no sign that Nash's unnatural calm was shaken" (p. 209).

4 A nice example of the necessity of appealing to the symbolic register so as to ascertain paternal authority is the "Divine Right of Kings." Being born into the position of a monarch is, in itself, apparently not enough to confer such authority. The prospective king or queen needs refer to God, or perhaps elaborate genealogical (that is, symbolic) lines of ascent. As always in Lacan, one can locate a Freudian precedent to his theorizing. In the case of the crucial role that the symbolic plays in securing paternity, we might refer to Freud's interest, in *Totem and Taboo* (1912–1913), with the totemic figures (and all the

associated symbolic rules and rituals) that made both clan identities and related effects of paternal authority possible.

5   As is perhaps obvious, this process does not always meet with success. The precise circumstances under which a delusion can take on such an organizational role and enable a psychotic subject to attain stabilization (a process conceptualized in Lacanian theory as that of "the delusional metaphor") remains an important area of research in the Lacanian tradition (see, for example, Lacan, 1993; Redmond, 2014; Vanheule, 2011, 2020; Ver Eecke, 2019).

6   The discourse of psychosis as madness/psychopathology is so pervasive that to even try and make the Lacanian position clear (namely, that psychosis, like neurosis, is a psychic structure that is not inherently psychopathological or "abnormal") is to risk further perpetuating detrimental stereotypes of psychosis. I have been tempted to suggest that Lacanian theory should risk a different nomenclature, referring to "subjects of foreclosure" rather than to "psychotics" simply so as to strike some distance from the pejorative associations that come with reference to "psychosis." (Foreclosure is considered by Lacanians to be the characteristic – indeed structural – defense mechanism that is defining of psychotic structure. Foreclosure, as such, can be considered as the primary underlying and essential feature, more elementary and crucial than any symptomatic features of psychosis).

References

American Psychiatric Association. (2013). *Diagnostic and statistical manual of mental disorders* (5th ed.). Washington, DC: Author.

Capps, D. (2003). John Nash's predelusional phase: A case of acute identity confusion. *Pastoral Psychology, 51*(5), 291–313.

Capps, D. (2004a). John Nash's delusional decade: A case of paranoid schizophrenia. *Pastoral Psychology, 52*(3), 193–218.

Capps, D. (2004b). John Nash's postdelusional period: A case of transformed narcissism. *Pastoral Psychology, 52*(4), 289–313.

Capps, D. (2005). John Nash: Three phases in the career of a beautiful mind. *Journal of Religious Health, 44*, 363–376.

Capps, D. (2011). John Nash, game theory, and the schizophrenic brain. *Journal of Religious Health, 50*, 145–162.

Evans, D. (1996). *An introductory dictionary of Lacanian psychoanalysis*. London: Routledge.

Freud, S. (1909). Analysis of a phobia in a five-year-old boy ('Little Hans') (1966–1974). In S. Freud (Ed.), *The standard edition of the complete psychological works of Sigmund Freud* (J. Strachey, Trans., Vol. 10, pp. 1–147). London: Hogarth.

Freud, S. (1911). Psycho-analytic notes on an autobiographical account of a case of paranoia (Dementia Paranoides) (1966–1974). In S. Freud (Ed.), *The standard edition of the complete psychological works of Sigmund Freud* (J. Strachey, Trans., Vol. 12, pp. 1–79). London: Hogarth.

Freud, S. (1912–1913). Totem and taboo: Some points of agreement between the mental lives of savages and neurotics (1966–1974). In S. Freud (Ed.), *The standard edition of the complete psychological works of Sigmund Freud* (J. Strachey, Trans., Vol. 13, pp. 1–161). London: Hogarth.

Freud, S. (1914). On narcissism: An introduction (1966–1974). In S. Freud (Ed.), *The standard edition of the complete psychological works of Sigmund Freud* (J. Strachey, Trans., Vol. 14, pp. 67–102). London: Hogarth.

Gabbard, G. (2014). *Psychodynamic psychiatry in clinical practice*. Washington, DC: American Psychiatric Publishing.

Hook, D. (2017). *Six moments in Lacan*. London & New York: Routledge.

Howard, R. (dir.). (2001). *A beautiful mind*. Dreamworks Picture. Universal Studios.

Kernberg, O. (1986). Factors in the treatment of narcissistic personalities. In A. P. Morrison (Ed.), *Essential papers on narcissism* (pp. 213–244). New York: New York University Press.

Kohut, H. (1966). Forms and transformations of narcissism. *Journal of the American Psychoanalytic Association, 14*, 243–272.

Lacan, J. (1993). *The psychoses. The seminar of Jacques Lacan: Book III*. London & New York: W.W. Norton.

Lacan, J. (2020). *The object relation. The seminar of Jacques Lacan: Book IV*. London: Polity Press.

Leader, D. (2011). *What is madness?* London: Penguin Putnam.

Leader, D. (2016). *Working with psychosis*. Lambeth and Southwark Mind Psychotherapy Clinic Launch. www.youtube.com/watch?v=OF8-9w2bPDw.

Lowen, A. (1983). *Narcissism: Denial of the true self*. New York: Palgrave Macmillan.

McWilliams, N. (2011). *Psychoanalytic diagnosis*. New York: Guildford Press.

Nash, J. (1994/2002). Autobiography. In H. W. Kuhn & S. Nasar (Eds.), *The essential John Nash* (pp. 5–11). Princeton, NJ: Princeton University Press.

Nasar, S. (1998). *A beautiful mind: The life of mathematical genius and Nobel laureate John Nash*. London & New York: Simon & Schuster.

Porter, R. (2003). *Madness: A brief history*. Oxford: Oxford University Press.

Redmond, J. D. (2014). *Ordinary psychosis and the body: A contemporary Lacanian approach*. London & New York: Palgrave Macmillan.

Rogers, A. (2016). *Incandescent alphabets*. London: Karnac Books.

Samels, M. (dir.). (2002). *A brilliant madness*. Yellow Jersey Films for American Experience. PBS. Home Video. (Written and Directed by Mark Samels).

Sass, L. (2017). *Madness and modernism: Insanity in the light of modern art, literature, and thought*. Oxford: Oxford University Press.

Scull, A. (2015). *Madness and civilization*. Princeton, NJ: Princeton University Press.

Vanheule, S. (2011). *The subject of psychosis: A Lacanian perspective*. London & New York: Palgrave Macmillan.

Vanheule, S. (2020). On a question prior to any possible treatment of psychosis. In D. Hook, C. Neill, & S. Vanheule (Eds.), *Reading Lacan's Ecrits: From 'the freudian thing' to 'remarks on Daniel Lagache'* (pp. 163–205). London & New York: Routledge.

Ver Eecke, W. (2019). *Breaking through schizophrenia: Lacan and Hegel for talk therapy*. London & New York: Rowman & Littlefield.

Wang, C. (2019). *Subjectivity in-between times: Exploring time in Lacan's work*. London & New York: Palgrave Macmillan.

Chapter 8

The touch from without/
the force from within

Ronald Schenk

ABSTRACT: This chapter explores the idea of madness as it appears in its foundations in psychiatry, philosophy, myth, anthropology, and literature. It starts
with the experience of a young man diagnosed with schizophrenia and treated
by Western psychiatry; an account which shows a long-standing cultural ambiva-
lence toward madness. We look to the Greeks, who revered a god of madness,
Dionysus; to Julian Jaynes's sense of Homeric culture as itself, "schizophrenic";
and to Plato's deliberation on the four forms of madness as a boon to humanity.
Shamans of native peoples will be seen to treat their patients through an experience akin to madness. The mad King Lear's speeches will be analyzed for their
own logic, indicating the Renaissance sensibility of madness as representing the
reality of the darkness of the human condition. We follow Foucault's footsteps in
his sense of madness as a construction relative to the context of societal values
and his exposition of the classical age as the turn toward the modern medicalization, separation, and confinement of madness in service to power. The humaniza-
tion in Pinel's approach leads eventually to the quest for meaning in madness by
Jung and Perry. Finally, the rites engaged by our initial patient with a native healer
in Africa will bring our exploration full circle.

KEYWORDS: confinement, cultural norms, madness, separation, shamanism

Franklin lost

Frank, a drug-free boy of mixed white and Black race, age 15, was lying in bed
one night, when he saw a square. He found he was able to go into the square, and
there, he encountered a circle with a spiral form protruding rays, which, in turn,
were bisected by another larger circle. Then the inner circle became something
like a sun, yellow and orange, and then a tunnel, glowing green and yellow, as
if by itself, creating a space down into which he could move. He came across
an opening and could see a pyramid and, behind it, columns on both sides. He
moved through them, finding himself 10 feet off the ground looking down on a

single open eye. Rising higher, he could see water glistening in sunlight and two jewels. Further on was another tunnel like a cave, shiny and full of colors. Then he fell asleep.

Frank had experienced something of a troubled childhood. Although testing out at a "genius" IQ level, he had a history of difficulties in school, was overly perfectionistic so that he couldn't concentrate well or finish his work, had chronic headaches and periodic rages, and found socializing a problem. His sense of self was fluid so that differentiation from others was a challenge. Periodically, he seemed to exist in a different world – one where he was intimately connected with animals and peoples of far-away cultures. At the same time, he was very artistic and musical, extraordinarily insightful regarding others' emotions and motivations, with an uncanny, at times prophetic, sense of timing. He was inquisitive about the world around him, very much taken with symbology, and was often expressive in an extraordinarily poetic way. Frank had written in his journal:

> Dissatisfaction with my life brings me into my own mind. There, I lose track of my heart which wants me to be boundless, searching, living, doing, succeeding, feeling. . . . Then, as if a guardian angel had a hand in my fate. I break free, in sacrifice, humility, devotion, or hatred, impudence, accident, or rage. Then I reawaken or resurrect.
>
> (Russell, 2014, p. 29)

Months after the described "vision," Frank had a mental "breakdown" during which he experienced delusions that his friends were out to kill him, suicidal command hallucinations, and depressive symptoms. He was hospitalized and treated with antipsychotic medications. Then followed years of encounters with the American medical establishment, in which context his experience was understood as reflecting a "disease." This approach utilizes psychotropic medications that can permanently alter mind and body through side effects such as tardive dyskinesia, obesity, and diabetes, often resulting in deterioration of brain function, and a general "zombification" of mind (Russell, 2014, pp. 81–82). In addition, there were revolving door cycles of hospitalizations oriented toward "symptom management," half-way houses organized around social control, and psychological counseling emphasizing "cognitive functioning" and "ego development" – in short, a maze of systems operating with varying degrees of "success" in meeting treatment goals, yet demonstrating no interest in the value of Franklin's actual experiences, forcing him into a mold centered around mainstream societal values.

Frank's condition is one that is experienced across cultures. Different peoples at different points in time display a range of attitudes and behaviors related to this state, which for the purpose of this chapter, we shall call "madness." Madness can be seen as that which lies outside the realm of the symbolic order held by the body politic, and it is considered by contemporary Western medicine as a disease of the mind, to be treated with medication aimed at reducing or eliminating symptoms considered as irrational. To the extent that a person experiencing madness is thought to be at risk for endangering self and others, they are excluded from community through hospitalization. Alternatively, the cultures of ancient Greece and those of contemporary Third World societies give indications that what modernity considers "mad" is actually an attunement with an entirely different consciousness that can be beneficial and is deserving of its own place in the community.

From a psycho-historical perspective, we can say that Frank and those who treated him have inherited a long and varied tradition regarding the relationship between reason and madness. This chapter will explore the tensions that emerge in this relationship in terms of what passes as culturally accepted order and its counterweight in the "disorders" of madness. The exploration will be oriented around the experience of madness in three figures beginning with Frank's initial encounter with Western psychiatry as previously described. The context of the Renaissance reveals a second example in Shakespeare's King Lear – famous for his "madness" but who, upon close scrutiny, in fact reveals a sensibility to his social environment that expresses its underbelly of deceit. Frank will be revisited, now with an entirely different experience of his process. This time, he is embedded within a non-Western ethos, and it is through the rituals of an African culture that he is eventually healed.

Using these examples of the experience of madness as touchstones, we shall make forays into various approaches to madness that illustrate vast differences of cultural assumptions and worldviews. These excursions will include the perspective that ancient Greek culture itself was schizophrenic during the Homeric period, the complexity of Platonic thought that considers madness as informing exceptional revered states of mind, the sensibility in some cultures that individuals who carry conditions that might be considered "schizophrenic" are able to become healers themselves through shamanic rituals, and the vision of madness by the mainstream Renaissance that madness holds a separate dark, tumultuous cosmic reality. The movement in the West to separate, confine, and medicalize madness will be traced from its roots in the Enlightenment to the present day, along with a slowly evolving counterpoint in the history of psychiatry that looks to madness as an aspect of personal evolution.

Schizophrenia as cultural norm

The history of madness and its treatment in the West coalesces around the tension between reason and madness, and their places in culture. The content and emphasis on each side shifts with changes in cultural ethos and milieu. Psychologist Julian Jaynes speculates that the subjective ordering, highly rational Western mind we know as modern consciousness evolved in the Greek world out of a cultural consciousness we would now consider to be "schizophrenic." Jaynes starts with the idea that consciousness is not the ordering, reasoning basis of conceptual experience we have come to think of it as. Rather consciousness is an operation, a way of "seeing" through analogy, a mode of creating a world. In other words, consciousness is generated through metaphor. This is an important insight because it enables madness to be seen as a structuring of signifiers that diverge with the mainstream of culture. Jaynes (1976) looks to Homeric man to develop a sense of daily life that was controlled by voices thought of as divinities. He sees in the *Iliad* an account of men acting, reacting, thinking, and feeling, not out of a subjective "I," but at the behest of gods.

> It is a god who . . . rises out of the grey sea and consoles (Achilles) in his tears of wrath on the beach by his black ships, a god who whispers low to Helen to sweep her heart with homesick longing, a god who hides Paris in a mist in front of the attacking Menelaus, a god who tells Glaucus to take bronze for gold.
>
> (p. 72)

For Jaynes, the voices of the gods were what we now refer to as hallucinations. He attributes this phenomenon to a predominance of right-brained activity in Homeric man, in which the right brain expressed itself through voices heard by the left brain as expressions from the divine world. Here we might say Jaynes is using physiology as a concretized metaphor for the idea that sanity and madness are two interrelated systems or orderings, the right brain with its basis in imagination and the left functioning out of reason.

Jaynes (1976) suggests that madness, with its "hallucinations and delusions" experienced as separate from "reason," only came about around 400 BC with the emergence of individual subjectivity.[1] Jaynes can be considered to be imaginatively stretching in his depiction of the collective consciousness of Homeric culture.[2] His ideas do, however, "normalize" schizophrenia in that they present an entire form of cultural consciousness that is based with what we would now call the unconscious.[3] The bicameral explanation further suggests a physiological connection between creativity and auditory hallucinations.

By comparison, classicist E.R. Dodds (1951) does attribute a "self" to Homeric man which differentiates between normal and abnormal behavior, the latter associated with divine agencies. All extreme feelings, thoughts, and actions – in short, the irrational aspects of the personality, or the *atai* – were attributed to gods. *Thumos* is an independent organ of feeling in the chest that informs us of needed action; *menos*, an upwelling of energy; *arete*, potency as a fighter. Any subjective experience that seems unaccountable or arrives as a spontaneous upwelling or a matter of *moira* or fate would be experienced as a presentation of a god. The *atai* is a form of punishment meant for those who have committed crimes. Examples include Prometheus, perpetually chained to a rock with his liver devoured each day by an eagle, only to be reformed anew every night; Antigone, buried alive for giving her brother funeral rites; and Orestes, pursued by the Furies for the murder of his mother. Sophocles (1960) expresses the terror evoked by the mad turbulence of punishing divinity:

> Fortunate they whose lives have no taste of pain.
> For those whose house is shaken by the gods
> Escape no kind of doom. It extends to all the kin
> Like the wave that comes when the winds of Thrace
> Run over the dark sea.
> The black sand of the bottom is brought from the depth;
> The beaten capes sound back with hollow cry.
>
> (ll 583 ff., p. 202)

In sum, the gods can be conceptualized as forces outside of human control that give shape to extreme forms of human experience that would be considered as madness in other cultural systems.

Shamanic culture

In non-Western cultures, those experiences that psychiatry is likely to conceptualize as "schizophrenia" are treated with an inclusive approach, and in many cases, the patient is considered a budding healer. In these cultures, one finds a communal, inclusive orientation, and aberrant behavior is contained and treated by the community. Individuals are cared for by empathic caregivers, given local natural medicines, and, most importantly, provided with space to recover in their own way. This enables the individual to become asymptomatic in less than half the time as those with similar conditions in industrialized countries (Banerjee, 2012). In cultures where healing is conducted by shamans, crises in individuals with psychotic-like experiences – hallucinations, delusions, seizures, hyper-reflexivity – are seen as calling for necessary separation from standard social structures. In these cultures, the individual is considered to be undergoing a calling to the vocation of shamanic healing (Esima, 2019). The individual is conducted into initiatory procedures by both established shamans and by what are held as tutelary "spirits." He or she then learns the healing arts which involve the capacity to enter other worlds, especially those of the offending spirits and the dead.

In the words of Mircea Eliade (1964), the budding shaman "is projected onto a vital plane that shows him the fundamental data of human existence, that is, solitude, danger, hostility of the surrounding world" (p. 27). In the ancient Greek culture, shamanic healing became the incubation rites of Asclepius wherein the patient would be visited by the Great Snake or the god that caused the disease, an encounter which in itself would bring about healing. We can see that madness in these cultures has a special meaning that involves a connection with a world outside of the predominate everyday structures of the culture – a connection which can be beneficial to the wider community.

Platonic madness

With Plato, we are firmly in the differentiated but interrelated sensibility of sanity and madness, the latter either caused by human ailments or by divine intervention. Paradoxically, the latter has greatest value in that it is via escape from the everyday mind in divine inspiration that one can remember the archetypal forms of true being. Through the voice of Socrates, Plato (1961) envisions this event in four conditions:

1   [I]n reality, the greatest blessings come by way of madness, indeed of mad-
     ness that is heaven sent. It was when they were mad that the prophetess at
     Delphi and the priestesses at Dodona achieved so much for which both states
     and individuals in Greece are thankful; when sane they did little or nothing
     (Phaedrus, 244a-b, p. 491).

Prophecy, governed by the god, Apollo, was considered the greatest of arts, enlist-
ing individuals conversant with the ways of the gods to offer guidance to those
suffering under conditions of unfathomable human dilemma. The two most notable Apolline prophets were the Sibyl and the Pythia, into each of whom the god
would enter using her vocal faculties as his own.

2   [W]hen grievous maladies and afflictions have beset certain families by reason
     of some ancient sin, madness has appeared among them, and breaking out into
     prophecy has secured relief. . . . Thus did madness secure, for him that was
     maddened aright and possessed, deliverance from his troubles (244e, p. 492).

Dionysus was "the mad god" whose sudden appearance caused individuals, particularly women, to become possessed and raving, inciting ecstatic savagery and
lust for blood, and generating devastation to human order through terror. In Euripides' play, the *Bacchae*, Dionysus can be seen as representing a force beyond
human reason and control. However paradoxical, this madness, when sublimated
into a ritual dance involving temporary abandonment and dissociation from
oneself, brought about a cathartic healing effect through the purgation of toxic
impulses, as well as the birth of theater.

3   There is a third form of madness of which the muses are the source. This
     seizes a tender, virgin soul and stimulates it to rapt passionate expression,
     especially in lyric poetry (245a, p. 492).

Poetic expression comes about as a madness induced by the grace of the Muses.
Poetry, as true speech, emerges as something outside of oneself given by the divine.

4   Mark . . . the fourth sort of madness . . . the best of all forms of divine posses-
     sion, both in itself and in its sources, both for him that has it and for him that
     shares therein – when he that loves beauty is touched by such madness, he is
     called a lover (249d, p. 496).

Erotic madness was inspired by Aphrodite and Eros. For Plato, it was the most valued of all divine possessions, in that it was the lover who was able to apprehend the beauty of the world, and through this apprehension was reminded of the true beauty of the heavenly forms. It was by the light of Aphrodite shining through all worldly things that humans were able to sense ultimate Being.

In Platonic philosophy, the rational mind searching for the truth of divine forms was always of the highest value. What Plato imagined as the blessings of madness were inspired by the divine and were seen as precursor conditions for the rational mind striving toward ultimate knowledge. The soul did encompass an irrational aspect in its passions, but the passions could be tamed and used in the energic striving for enlightenment. The rational and the irrational, the pursuit of transcendent forms of being as truth, and the possession by otherness were ultimately seen as aspects of the same process. In sum, Plato held that there is an irrational part of the soul, the passions, that in themselves are detrimental, but which are subject to beneficial adjustment through the rational mind. Greek thought of the 4th century BC came to hold that there are different kinds of madness – the inspirational and the toxic – with the latter still subject to transformation into beneficial agency.

In summary, in both antiquity and in contemporary non-industrialized cultures, we see an attitude toward madness which posits it as a condition of separation from familiar identity which is produced through the effect of an external superhuman influence. This phenomenon is considered to be an aspect of the natural workings of the psyche that is connected to a realm outside of the common ground of the culture.

King Lear: the first mad patient

The French philosopher Michel Foucault (1973) traced the history of the turn in the Western imagination regarding madness from its place in the Middle Ages, when it was seen as a form of possession by devils, through the Renaissance, when it served as a kind of touchstone to another world of disorder and death. Foucault notes that by the end of the Middle Ages, leprosy had all but vanished in Europe and, by the Renaissance, its place was taken by madness. The figure of the leper representing a disease of moral values was replaced by the figure of the fool/madman, carried in the image of the Ship of Fools loaded with madmen eternally seeking, as if in search of the peace of mind offered by Renaissance Humanism. Pictured in a kind of ghost ship, madness was exiled, yet kept vividly in the imagination, able to appear spontaneously with the burst of the winds, close enough to be visualized in the harbor but safely moored at the threshold of community in a liminal space.

The proximity of water in relation to madness suggests not only a purifying quality, but the dynamics of its process: cast out on the sea with its limitless possibilities of tumultuous conditions; passage across a surging chaotic, dark, and deadly disorder; and ambivalent arrival only to set sail once more. The Ship of

Fools represents folly as a mocking of existence involving the whole of humanity in complicit understanding of its blindness and helplessness in the ironic face of nothingness laughing at the fallacy of power, the deceit of knowledge and wisdom, and the meaninglessness of suffering. Foucault (1973) writes

> On all sides, madness fascinates man. . . . When a man deploys the arbitrary nature of his madness, he confronts the dark necessity of the world; the animal that haunts his nightmares and his nights of privation is his own nature, which will lay bare hell's pitiless truth.

(p. 23)

Foucault concludes his discussion on the Renaissance with several examples in which madness became a commonplace spectacle, the most important for the purposes of this chapter being the madness of desperate passion in King Lear, where madness is seen as the irony and paradox of a life turned upside down, becoming the darkened light of truth in its severity and harshness.

We can now turn to King Lear as a paradigmatic figure in our presentation of madness as a condition caught between two symbolic worlds – that of reason in quest for power and control, and the metaphorical in search of underlying reality. Shakespeare (1952) constructed his play around several aspects of the central tension between reason and madness. Nature is presented as part of an order given in man through birth versus that which is man-made and therefore subject to human defects. Nature is also an intergenerational order based on loyal affection versus nature as a fundamental disorder of cosmic forces characterized by violence and the animalistic struggle for survival. Self-aggrandizement is ultimately revealed as a kind of madness in relation to authentically loving human relationship. Vision as knowledge, especially self-knowledge, serves as a rock of reason in contrast to blindness of self as mad folly. The possession of "all" is madness in relation to the grounded need for "nothing." The irrationality that one uncovers as "home" contrasts to the fundamental reality of the human condition in homelessness. In sum, the unique psychological aspect of these tensions is how paradoxically they play into each other such that what seems mad is in fact real and vice-versa: the Fool expresses wisdom in his jokes; Cordelia gives Lear everything when she says she has "nothing"; punishment of the body clarifies the mind; Gloucester finally "sees" when he is literally blinded; it is in the ultimate violence of inner madness and outer storm that human order based on humility and love can take its form. The play can be understood as a necessary mad journey through these tensions – the release of home as domain, the treachery of filial disloyalty, the rage of perceived injustice, madness and self-dismemberment in the stripping away of all layers of man-made accoutrement down to literal flesh and bone which manifests the ultimate image of self and the human condition.

What follows is a psychoanalysis of the "madness" of Lear. Act III finds the king and his fool alone on a barren heath in the midst of a violent storm. Lear, having given away his domain to two of his daughters in exchange for their deceitful vows of love, finds himself rejected by them, discharged from house and home, and stripped of all acknowledgment of kingship and fatherhood. The entire scene is an image of the human condition as a form of madness – alone in a stark landscape accompanied only by folly, beset by the violence of nature. The outer storm matches the inner storm of Lear's rage, which has been building with each sign of rejection by his daughters. He curses the natural structure of human generation and relationship. Although it seems mad to be in this place without shelter, ironically, Lear has found his home and a form of sanity in the place where inner and outer meet; as opposed to the castle of deceit wherein true madness lies, the tempest of mind serving as an appropriate response to the betrayal of filial ingratitude, deceit, and violent hostility.

The following scene takes place in a hovel occupied by a nobleman, the loyal Gloucester's son, Edgar, disguised as a madman to save himself from the treachery of his brother – madness as the only sane recourse in the face of an irrational human order. Lear sees in Edgar's feigned mad condition the essence of the human condition and tears off his clothes as the last vestiges of human order. He proclaims, "Is man no more than this? . . . . thou art the thing itself. Unaccommodated man is no more but such a poor, bare, forked animal as thou art" (III, iv, ll., p. 106–112). Together with a loyal servant, Kent, who is also disguised, having been banished for his honesty, the Fool, and Edgar acting as if mad, Lear subsequently conducts a mock trial of his daughters in striving for an imaginative rectification of their injustice. Although he is madly identified with the psycho-dramatic exposition, his viewpoint accurately cuts through the façade of the daughters' deceit, and he is showing that he "sees" them and is creating justice for himself in the only way possible – through a fantasy of the institution of justice. Here, among figures who in various ways survive by disguising the truth, what is considered "mad" is objectively real.

Lear then sinks further into a fantastical realm, that is yet reflective of reality in its own way. He is, in his loyal daughter Cordelia's words, "mad as the vexed sea," as he appears crowned with wildflowers and weeds. This clown-like dress can be seen as Lear's mocking of nature and the curse he feels from its order. His ensuing mad speech has a coherent logic, reflective in its own way of Lear's reality. We might seek to psychoanalyze the speech line by line to reveal the reality it portrays through metaphor (my interpretation offered in italics):

- "[T]hey cannot touch me for coining, I am the King himself;"

  As king, it is his natural right to power as represented by coining money.

- "Nature's above art in that respect. There's your press money."

  The right to fight for and distribute power as represented in giving money to soldiers cannot be usurped through contrived artifice.

- "That fellow handles his bow like a crowkeeper, draw me a soldier's yard."

  Lear's mind goes from his station of sovereignty to the battle that has been raging inside. The archer is like a scarecrow and he pulls the string of his bow back a full yard.

- "Look, look, a mouse."

  As we saw in his encounter with Edgar, in his madness, Lear has come to see human being in its essence as no more significant than that of the lowest animal. At Cordelia's death, he will be pitting human life against that of dog, horse, and rat.

- "There's my gauntlet, I'll prove it on a giant. Bring up the brown bills."

  Now back to the battle with his sons-in-law through armed challenge and the call to the infantry.

- "Oh, well-flown bird! I' the clout, I' the clout. Hewgh!"

  The image of the archer; he has hit the target with the accompanying whiz of the arrow – a metaphor for his hitting the target of truth.

                                                                    (IV, vi, 83–92)

Lear goes on to rage against his daughters and the very act of copulation which gives rise to such offspring. However, he becomes calmed with the recognition of the blinded Gloucester, who arrives having been led by his son disguised as a madman, "the mad leading the blind," a mirror reflection of Lear's own suffering and his sense of order turned upside down. Gloucester confesses he can only see the world "feelingly," and Lear responds, "What, art mad? A man may see how this world goes with no eyes. Look with thine ears" (IV, vi, 153–4), and *see* how justice becomes interchanged with the thief, thus the dog ends up on the throne of authority. The observing Edgar can only wonder, "Oh, matter and impertinency mixed! Reason in madness!" (IV vi, 178–9). Lear ultimately declares himself the jovial king, the figure of life itself which can only be caught by running, and runs out, madness as living metaphor for life's unpredictable movement.

In summary, through his encounter with the underworld of madness Lear has come to "know" (one of the first words he utters in the play) himself in his humble essence, the true king, and to come to a sensibility of the human condition as essentially seething with madness. By divesting himself of home, land, the accoutrements of social life, and even the natural order of intergenerational loyalty, the paradoxical reality is revealed that nothing is more irrational than the rational order, "the great stage of fools," conceived by man in conjunction with the natural order of the cosmos. Madness then becomes its own language, a system of metaphors known through feeling in a storm of interaction signifying to the world a different reality – one that does not lend itself to rational order, control, certainty, or authorization. The internal/external storm of madness in the play takes us back to the Greek sense of man at the mercy of the gods; "As flies to wanton boys are we to the gods" (IV ii, 37). It is the mad fury of the gods that is seen as the punishing force. This also resonates with Plato's sense of the need for "madness" in order to step outside of the common mind to sense the eternal forms of reality. Likewise, Lear's descent and confrontation with his phantom protagonists is reminiscent of the shaman's journey into a transcendent realm to battle the antagonist spirits. As with shamanism, it is this mad encounter that brings about ultimate healing and reconstitution.

Madness behind walls

In what he terms "the classical period," Foucault notes a shift in attitude toward madness. Whereas in the Middle Ages, madness was seen as a manifestation of demonic possession (indicative of sin in need of cathartic purgation), and in the Renaissance, madness was the wandering signifier of the continuous threat of a dark beyond, in the 17th century, madness was hijacked as an outlaw "other" and thus consigned to confinement. The hospital now served as a wall of concealment and a container for establishing the authority and control of reason. Madness became medicalized and measured against the judgment of reason's orientation toward economics, which lead "madness" to be intrinsically tied to morality. Idleness becomes a sin in a world where productivity and usefulness are primary virtues. The poor, unemployed, criminal, and insane were then housed out of sight in a space regulated for optimum control and militaristic order. Foucault (1973) writes:

> confinement conceals both a metaphysics of government and a politics of religion; it is situated, as an effort of tyrannical synthesis, in the vast space separating the garden of God and the cities which men, driven from paradise, have built with their own hands. The house of confinement in the classical age constitutes the densest symbol of that "police" which conceived of itself as the civil equivalent of religion for the edification of a perfect city.
>
> (p. 63)

For Foucault, the bourgeois order, founded in the mindset of reason, understood madness as connoting a scandal giving rise to the odor of shame – on the one hand, around its perceived bestiality and frenzy and, on the other, around its lackadaisical withdrawal from the rhythm of economic production. Whereas in the Renaissance, human animality was linked to the protection of nature, it now becomes subject to correction through discipline. While withdrawal had been associated to habitation at the edge of the human condition and its storms, it now becomes idleness to be brutalized into productivity. In sum, madness is now seen through a lens of remedial action.

Passion and imagination, associated with madness, come under prosecutorial scrutiny. Foucault (1973) quotes Francois Sauvages:

> The distraction of our mind is the result of our blind surrender to our desires, our incapacity to control or to moderate our passions. Whence these amorous frenzies . . . this melancholy which is caused by grief . . . these indispositions, these corporeal vices which cause madness, the worst of all maladies.
>
> (p. 85)

Passion is regarded as not only providing a platform for violence in its careening toward frenzy, but also renders genuine repose inaccessible in that passion can turn against itself, evoking insurmountable conflict and contradiction. Foucault continues quoting Sauvages: "It is not unheard of that the passions, being very violent, generate a kind of tetanus or catalepsy such that the person then resembles a statue more than a living being" (p. 90).

In the grip of passion, the unity of body and soul begins to fragment, and an irrational movement occurs in which imagination takes over from reason. Fragments become reality and the immediate image obtains a disproportionate value, becoming itself the whole truth. In other words, an immediate experience or idea gains the sense of ultimate truth through passion, gathering to it others until this complex becomes the center of an absurd unity of consciousness. A scenario might run as follows: an imagined guilt produces a fear of accusation leading to a terror of prosecution, finally resulting in a fantasy of imprisonment. Self-blinding madness is now associated with passion, in conjunction with imagination, in service to a false freedom which culminates in a disastrous confiscation and envelopment of reason by madness. Foucault (1973) observes:

> Being both error and sin, madness is simultaneously impurity and solitude; it is withdrawn from the world, and from truth; but it is by that very fact imprisoned in evil. Its double nothingness is to be the visible form of that non-being which is *evil*, and to utter in the void and in the sensational appearances of its delirium, the non-being of error.
>
> (pp. 175–176)

The state, in service to reason, now takes over a regime of correction for this error in rationality by means of confinement. Medical treatment is at once a moral and metaphysical corrective in bringing about adaptation to the society of reason. Since body and soul are interrelated entities, techniques are applied to the body as treatment of the soul: procedures of bleeding, purging, and blistering are applied. Iron is given to instill vigor and correct inherent weakness. Vinegar is utilized to purify the thickening of blood. Immersion in cold water dissolves dryness of spirit. Imposed regulation of movement as well as music brings the agitated and frenzied soul into harmony with the rhythm of the world ordered through reason.

By the end of the 17th and into the 18th centuries, the predominant cultural attitude toward madness turned to fear. In an age emphasizing liberty and the break away from immediate need, the madness of unlimited appetite took the form of cultural "shadow," with madness as the language of desire unhinged from reason. Foucault (1973) writes:

> liberty, far from putting man in possession of himself, ceaselessly alienates him from his essence and his world; it fascinates him in the absolute exteriority of other people and of money, in the irreversible interiority of passion and unfulfilled desire.
>
> (p. 214)

The air of liberty had loosened madness from its confines, and it came to represent everything that was a break from the shackles of the natural order. A compensatory response was expressed in the birth of the asylum – the walled retreat where madness could be observed and judged continuously. Now separated from the poor and the criminal and aligned in orderly blocks of cells under the ever-present scrutiny of authority, the restraint of madness became the imposition of guilt. Meaningless work acted as punishment for sin and instilled the habit of labor. The mad were considered as children to be kept under constant observation by officials acting as parents, thereby establishing an internal and external structure according to the social morality of the bourgeoise family. Foucault relates how a hysterical woman, drawn to destructive acts against self and environment, was in a state such that the director:

> in order to impress a feeling of terror upon her, spoke to her with the most energetic firmness, but without anger, and announced to her that she would henceforth be treated with the greatest severity. . . . Her repentance was announced by a torrent of tears which she shed for almost two hours.
>
> (p. 268)

The treatment was successful, the triumph for authority complete; the recognition of her guilt announced through the cascade of tears.

Foucault suggests that the view of madness in the classical period, seen at once as social crime and an error in reason, sets the stage for that of ensuing generations. Confinement removed the lacunae in reason from the social order, ironically enacting a kind of repression that was the hallmark of madness itself. The tolerance of the Renaissance became a mode of corrective action in the classical age in service to morality and economic order, resulting in confinement for the sake of control and systematic physical and emotional assaults. It was this medical format, geared toward regulation, that now can be seen as the foundation for the contemporary approach of psychiatry with the walls of the asylum giving way to the stultifying effects of psychotropic medication.

The post-classical period would see the inauguration of an alternative movement away from strict confinement behind asylum walls to what was seen as a
more humanistic approach. Foucault, however, considered this as just another
form of patriarchal control over the individual in the guise of empathy, but continuing to serve the needs of authority. Such as the case may be, we now leave
Foucault to follow the thread of this alternate approach, which will take us ultimately to a radically different orientation toward madness.

Meaning in madness

In the late 18th century and early 19th century, the French physician Phillippe
Pinel became the director of an institution in which he drastically modified the
approach of his predecessors with what he termed "moral therapy." Pinel made
the first description of the condition which would later be called by various names
leading up to the diagnosis of "schizophrenia." Although he instituted a strict
atmosphere, he also saw his patients as human beings with unique psychological features and histories. He relieved them of their chains and approached them
through conversation.

Pinel believed that healing could evolve from within the personality, and his
interventions were tailored to individual requirements, sensitive to the conflict
he saw between the need for dignity and the chaos of overpowering emotions.
Punishment was de-emphasized in favor of a firm opposition to delusional beliefs,
and the asylum staff was carefully trained. Many former patients later served as
employees. With his focus on individuality and his beliefs about the richness of
interior life, language as therapeutic, and healing as a natural process, Pinel can be
seen as a forbearer of future alternative approaches to madness.

In the late 19th century, the Burgholzli asylum in Zurich became a center for
advanced thinking in the research and treatment of schizophrenia. Auguste Forel
took over a corrupt and ill managed institution and initiated changes in accord-
ance with his humanitarian and socialist beliefs. He emphasized community living and the participation of both patients and staff in everyday maintenance work.
His successor, Eugene Bleuler, carried on this tradition. Heavily influenced by
Sigmund Freud, Bleuler saw the unconscious at work in schizophrenia (a term
he coined), and following Pinel, saw schizophrenia as a condition of splitting
between the mind and the emotions. His treatment laid emphasis on the consideration of symptoms as meaningful psychological expressions.

Bleuler's work was complemented and extended by his pupil and associate,
C.G. Jung. Through his use of the word association test, Jung came to understand psychopathology along the lines of Freud – a manifestation of unconscious
complexes – feeling-toned images formed into clusters of ideas which became
associated with similar experiences and when split off from ego control would
take on an energy that could dominate the ego. Through his work with schizophrenia, Jung at first considered psychopathology in terms of a compensating healing

function of the unconscious in relation to consciousness. However, as an aspect of his split from Freud, he soon came to see psychotic symptoms as having meanings beyond personal experience; rather, they were the manifestations of inherited images representing universal tendencies in human experience that he referred to as archetypes. He likened these symbolic expressions to the dreams of nonclinical individuals, especially "big dreams" carrying mythological motifs. In short, Jung was in effect giving schizophrenia a special place in the collective psychology – a parallel to shamanic practices, with schizophrenia being seen as an expression of universal psychological themes in the form of mythical images.

The work of John Weir Perry in the mid-20th century extended Jung's vision. Perry treated the acute psychotic process in young adults in a fashion completely contrary to the medical model of reducing symptoms through medication. Instead, in his treatment facilities and in the attitudes of his staff who were lay volunteers, he gave room for a process of psychic reconstitution to take place. Following mythical themes, Perry (1976) saw psychic breakdown in these individuals as part of a natural process on the part of the psyche to reorganize itself out of a condition of self-alienation. For Jung, each psyche has its own autonomous intention toward an essential unique being. The psychotic process was the psyche's way to completely dissolve itself for the purpose of reconfiguration in a reconstituted structure following universal mythical themes of psychological breakdown and renewal. Perry's (1974) therapeutic approach, without direction or previous assumptions of socialization, was to listen with curiosity and interest to the patient's affective imagery of delusions and hallucinations in an attempt to enter the patient's world. He regarded the primary need of the patient to be the expression of the imagery of their experience and for meaning to be found in this.

Perry brings us back to Plato's sensibility that the highest calling of the soul is to loosen itself from earth-bound logic and to follow the reason of a higher order. In his approach to treatment, he has also brought us back to the shamanic milieu of native cultures, in which the shaman takes an imaginary journey to another world to encounter the spirits of the disease and then return renewed.

Franklin regained

After several years of struggling though the morass of medication regimentations and controlling living situations that Western health services often provide for individuals in Frank's situation, Franklin's father, Dick, made a significant move. Dick, who had accompanied Frank through the years as a well-intended but uncomprehending caretaker, took him on a trip to Africa to view an annual migration of wildlife. The destination of this journey was especially important because a major theme in Frank's identity confusion had to do with his Black heritage. One night in a room at a farm for travelers, Frank had a breakthrough. He entered a psychic space with his attentive father in which he was able to express in a direct way for the first time his ambivalent feelings regarding his experience of his father through the years – controlling, not understanding, inferior in many ways. His thought process included his sense of association to, and in some cases identification with, symbolic images and themes which gave him a feeling of power in relation to his father. Prominent among these was that of the serpent, an archetypal symbol of healing and of the psychological underworld of irrationality that the Greeks would elicit in their ancient incubation healing rites. Russell (2014) recounts Frank's monologue:

> You've been making use of my information for the whole trip. For the wrong thing. You take my blood in the car and ingest it for the idea of being more powerful. That's what I think you are doing. . . . I know history in ways you do not. Where I go, the snake has been. Sixteen years after Park School, then I become the Snake King.
>
> (p. 195)

His calculation was correct; it had been 16 years since his graduation. Throughout the ensuing period, Frank had been struggling with identity issues relating to race. Having a white father and a Black mother, he had been unable to come to terms with his racial heritage living in a predominately white society. Now in the ancestral homeland of his black heritage, he was feeling empowered to confront his white father with feelings of being controlled and undermined. At the same time, Frank was identifying with both a personal and an archetypal symbol of power and healing. In third grade, a drawing of his alluded to the importance of the snake. In effect, the meaning of the image was speaking through Frank's voice:

> I'm a very strong man. I'm tired yeah, not much energy. I might die tomorrow, I don't know. Whoever was in Africa replaced my head. If the "Year of the Snake" was my brother as Genghis, I don't know.[4] . . Africa said I came here 16,000 years ago. It's subliminal and people don't believe it's true. . . . I'm just here suffering right now. I've been dunked, lowered, guinea'd into a position here in Africa. . . . If you want to be a guide, be a snake at the end of my lifetime. . . . Why don't you take your mask off? It seems as though you have been undermining me for years.
>
> (pp. 198–199)

Father and son were engaged in a painful, ruthlessly honest dialogue, with the son asserting his power by confronting the father on his failures, and the father owning up to his sense of failure, allowing himself to be openly vulnerable to his feelings of helplessness. Here an archetypal transformation can be seen to have taken place – the son "killing" the father in a necessary act of self-empowerment, while at the same time, the father gives up his hold on the station of authority. The relationship was now being conducted with an honesty that neither had previously experienced. The weight of the "craziness" inherent in the false relationship that

Franklin had lived with as his dis-ease became relieved. Son became father, a guide to his father who now became a neophyte. Power roles had been reversed. Because his father had courageously entered the "other" world of the son and received its reality, the son was now able to achieve a more authentic identity and to spend the trip and the ensuing months feeling more related to the world.

Upon their return from Africa, Dick went back over Frank's old writings and saw in them a genuine poetic capacity. In addition, he eventually discovered an internationally renowned African shaman to treat Frank. This man, Malidoma Somé, was able to see in Frank, an exceptional personality struggling to strad-dle two completely different psychological realms – to dwell in two homes, the spiritual and the material, in the way of a true shaman. In addition to his making his way in the everyday world of contemporary Western culture, Frank now could find a place with a mentor who could recognize his capability in a symbolic realm with its own logic. Dick's task as a father was not only to respect this experience, but to help Frank as much as possible to adapt to the mainstream world. Frank now had an ongoing relationship with a representative of the sha-manic world and an improved relationship with his father as a guide and support in everyday life.

Several months after Dick and Frank returned to the United States, Malidoma suggested another trip to Africa to work with a particular holy man or shaman he felt would have the capability to further heal Frank through his rituals. This was to be a family event, in which Frank and both his father and mother would take part. Malidoma's continuing sense was that Frank needed to have various chan-nels in his body/psyche cleared of the effects of adversaries in the form of various treatments of Western medicine which only blocked Frank's essential path. This "way" had to do with Frank's particular capacity to know two different worlds – the literal world of his Western culture and the symbolic world of his ancestors.

The trip was undertaken, and a "second opinion" from a stick diviner confirmed the gist of Malidoma's diagnosis. The diviner saw Frank as having been born under a particularly bright star, the light of which was difficult for the world of his family and community to hold so that his "adversaries," the practitioners of Western medicine, needed to divert its "glow" in different ways. This diagnosis is very much in keeping with Perry's idea that madness is the necessary response to an environmental impediment to the individuating process involved in a person's becoming a true self.

The various rituals were conducted over several days in the context of a group of individuals, but with Frank receiving particular attention. They consisted of holding sacred animals such as chickens and goats, and objects such as eggs, giv-ing prayers which were focused upon the idea of knowing what is sought after, and rubbing the animals and objects on the body. A liquid concoction of roots, herbs, and other ingredients boiled down and taken from a special clay vessel served as medicine to counter the effects of Western psychotropic medication. The sacred animals were sacrificed, with the chicken and hen needing to fall a certain way on their backs for their power to be effective. The climactic ritual was the sacrifice and ingestion of a bull, the most powerful of domestic animals, a ritual conducted with accompanying prayers and ceremony. The major thrust of the entire process for Frank was to terminate his Western medication, which was being gradually reduced, while at the same time, realigning his psyche to comport with his more essential nature.

We can see this enterprise both in form and content as a metaphorical event of symbolic enactment reflecting Perry's psychotherapeutic approach to schizophrenia. A diagnosis is made and a course of treatment prescribed, wherein the goal is one of identity formation which includes integrating an important part of the psyche which has been consigned to the unconscious. The prayers are reflective of the patient's monologue which takes place in psychotherapy, and which Frank spontaneously undertook with his father on their previous African trip. The contact with animals and objects and the imbibing of the liquid was a form of connecting with and integrating of sources of strength to the self. The particular discipline of the ritual was that everything had to be accomplished according to a certain regiment. If it wasn't, the operation would need to be repeated. This is reflective of the spiral pattern in a psychotherapeutic endeavor in which there is a constant back and forth processing between progressive integration and the forces of resistance in the patient's psyche.

Since this second "homecoming" to Africa and the therapeutic encounter with shamanic ritual forces, Frank has continued to forge a life for himself. He remained on his Western medication, but at a greatly reduced dosage without the severe side effects that he had previously suffered. He returned to living in group home circumstances, still with up and down days emotionally, but able to relate in a more direct way, to show an inherent warmth and humor in his relationships, to maintain a job, and to engage in a wide range of artistic pursuits.

Notes

1 Jaynes (1976) considers subjectivity to be a result of: "1) . . . the advent of writing; 2) the . . . fragility of hallucinatory control; 3) the unworkableness of gods in the chaos of historical upheaval; 4) the positing of internal cause in the observation of difference with others; 5) the acquisition of narrative . . . 6) the survival value of deceit; 7) a modicum of natural selection" (p. 221).
2 There are two references in the *Odyssey* that refer to craziness as a condition separate from normality – Polyphemus's screaming that "No-man" is trying to kill him is attributed to a "sickness," albeit from Zeus (9.410), and the disguised Odysseus is referred to as "knocked out of his senses" (18.327).
3 James Hillman follows Plato's idea (1961, "Symposium"), "Gentlemen I need hardly say that each god must command our homage" (180 e, p. 535), and writes (2007) that the gods are expressions of distinct energy fields or archetypes which include pathologies, "Each god is a way in which we are shadowed" (p. 35, n. 6), while Jung (1967) directly states, "The gods have become diseases." (p. 37).
4 Genghis Khan had taken his last journey during the Chinese year of the Snake.

References

Banerjee, A. (2012). Cross-cultural variance of schizophrenia in symptoms, diagnosis, and treatment. *Georgetown University Journal of Health Sciences, 6,* 18–24.

Dodds, E. R. (1951). *The Greeks and the irrational.* Berkeley: University of California Press.

Eliade, M. (1964). *Shamanism: Archaic techniques of ecstasy.* Princeton, NJ: Princeton University Press.

Esima, G. E. (2019). From sick to gifted: Discovering shamanic illness. In M. Brown & M. C. Charles (Eds.), *Women and psychosis: Multidisciplinary perspectives.* Lanham, MD: Lexington Books.

Foucault, M. (1973). *Madness and civilization: A history of insanity in the age of reason* (R. Howard, Trans.). New York: Vintage.

Hillman, J. (2007). *Mythic figures.* Putnam, CT: Spring Publications.

Jaynes, J. (1976). *The origin of consciousness in the breakdown of the bicameral mind.* Boston, MA: Houghton Mifflin.

Jung, C. (1967). *Alchemical studies: The collected works of C.G. Jung* (R.F.C. Hull, Trans., Vol. 13, 35, n. 7). Princeton, NJ: Princeton University Press.

Perry, J. (1974). *The far side of madness.* Eaglewood Cliffs, NJ: Prentice-Hall.

Perry, J. (1976). *Roots of renewal in myth and madness: The meaning of psychotic episodes.* San Francisco: Jossey-Bass.

Plato. (1961). Phaedrus, 265a. In E. Hamilton & H. Cairns (Eds.), *The collected dialogues of Plato* (R. Hackforth, Trans.). Princeton, NJ: Princeton University Press.

Plato. (1961). Symposium 180e. In E. Hamilton & H. Cairns (Eds.), *The collected dialogues of Plato* (M. Joyce, Trans.). Princeton, NJ: Princeton University Press.

Russell, D. (2014). *My mysterious son.* New York: Skyhorse.

Shakespeare, W. (1952). *The complete works* (G. B. Harrison, Ed.). New York: Harcourt, Brace and World.

Sophocles. (1960). Antigone. In D. Greene & R. Lattimore (Eds.), *Greek tragedies* (E. Wyckoff, Trans., Vol. 1). Chicago, IL: University of Chicago Press.

Chapter 9

Creative transformations

The establishment, the mystic, and the aesthetic drive

Marilyn Charles

ABSTRACT: There is a preciousness and a precariousness in individual potential. We come into the world utterly dependent upon those around us to keep us safe enough that we can develop our potential. However, for those driven by aesthetic or spiritual inspiration, normative elements in family and culture can prove deadening. The artist is, to some extent, dependent on others to support their projects, and yet, even the most gifted artists may not be recognized for their talents; what we would term "genius" is often a function of a perspective that is outside the bounds of consensual reality, such that, at times, the pursuit of creative endeavors can become profoundly lonely and even seem to take the form of a type of madness. Bion helps us to recognize the inevitable tensions between the establishment and the new idea, what he terms the mystic, who speaks back to us in an alien voice. How we listen to such voices without further alienating and driving the person into silence or madness remains a worthy challenge, so that we can preserve, protect, and nourish the very creativity we need in order to thrive.

KEYWORDS: madness, creativity, primary process, spirituality, Bion, Kristeva, Lacan

Much has been written about the uneasy line between psychosis and creativity. It may be that precisely what makes for a particularly unique artistic expression comes from an anomalous vantage point that can also make life arduous and painful (see, for example, Charles, 2010a; Charles & Telis, 2014). Being able to reference one's own unique sensibilities is inherent in the creative process. Indeed, Milner (1987) suggests that any work of art is "an externalization, through its shapes, lines and colors, of the unique psychophysical rhythm of the person making it" (p. 230). Finding one's own internal rhythms can require a great deal of solitude, and yet, too much isolation can leave one lost and alone (Green, 1972). At the extreme, creativity has been linked to madness and to psychotic illness, leading artists, at times, to avoid either art-making or the type of meaning-making invited by insight-oriented psychotherapies. In contrast to such polarized positions, investigators have found a common substrate that appears to underlie not only creativity and psychosis, but also mystical experience. This factor has been termed *transliminality*, in reference to the crossing of a threshold inherent in each of these phenomena (Thalbourne & Delin, 1999). Transliminality is linked with fantasy proneness and absorption, suggesting "susceptibility to, and awareness of, large volumes of imagery, ideation and affect – these phenomena being generated by subliminal, supraliminal and/or external input" (Thalbourne et al., 1997, p. 305).

This mode of apprehending experience aligns rather closely with what Sigmund Freud (1900) termed *primary process*, also termed *symmetrical logic* by Matte-Blanco (1975). In Matte-Blanco's framework, there is an appreciation for the differing ways of constructing meaning that come from the more primary, embodied, nonverbal knowledge structures versus the more logical, cognitive, rational systems. Where learning tends to be driven by experience, kinesthetic structures can be useful in holding the complexity of being human (Charles, 2010b). I have often turned to myth and literature as a way of contextualizing the human struggles I encounter in my life and in my clinical work (Charles, 2015). In some ways, this is a function of my difficulty in thinking from the category to the experience. Rather, I seem to be hopelessly embodied, moving from the experience to the articulation. Thus, the language of story speaks more directly to the place from which I come.

I began life somewhat myopic, which left me, I think, focusing on details and missing the larger picture. That type of focus was also useful in a family where isolation and unlinking each afforded a welcome refuge from pain. I found myself early on searching through literature for the meanings that eluded me, carried by inchoate sensibilities that alternately tormented and soothed me. Whereas in literature, I found kindred spirits to accompany me, it was in psychoanalytic writings that I began to find a conceptual map for the patterns of being and becoming that otherwise were too easily obscured by content. Learning, for example, about the intergenerational transmission of trauma has helped me make sense of the child I was and the woman I became. The desperation that undergirded my devalued attempts toward creative expression and engagement largely foundered those efforts, making even successes largely invisible and unsatisfying to me, disappearing like dust as the emotion fades.

That history has left me resonant to similar suffering in others, those who are left – or thrust – outside the gates. Levinas (1999) marks the ethical imperative lodged in the call from the suffering in the human face. I link that call to a memory I have from watching films made by attachment researcher Stephen Suomi (2011) of the avoidantly-attached young apes who were caught in the wilderness between the childhood home from which they had been evicted and the impossibility of finding a new home, given what they had failed to learn that might have enabled that transition. I see that suffering in those I work with who have been pushed outside the gates by family and social structure, left to suffer in a wilderness that seems endless and almost unendurable. Structurally, I see their dilemma in the terms that Lacan referred to as the psychotic position, through this language recognizing that the experience of being left outside shapes the individual in a process of abjection (Kristeva, 1982; Vanheule, 2011).

Recognition of the force of abjection and marginalization in the etiology of what we have come to term *psychotic disorders*, individuals in northern Finland have developed what they term the *Open Dialogue Method* (Seikkula et al., 2006). Based on a humanistic, person-centered approach to human struggles, teams of health providers go into the home of families where an individual is suffering from a psychotic break and talk with the sufferer and the family members about the problems they are encountering. In the process of listening, talking, formulating, and respectfully engaging with one another, the affective intensity within the family is attenuated and family members are invited to more effectively think about their dilemmas. If you think about what we know about mirror neurons (Gallese, 2009), it makes sense that providing an experience of reflective, thoughtful engagement helps to set such a process in place whereby the sufferer and family members are provided models of reflective thought and effective problem solving.

In my own work, I find that, particularly with such persons, being able to work with the family, as well as the individual, is an incredible gift, bringing into vivid relief the interpersonal dilemmas at play. That frame of reference in even one case helps us to take seriously and try to think and feel our way into speech that can otherwise sound odd, metaphoric, or even inconceivable. That type of experience can also help us recognize ways in which what seems inconceivable can be a function of our defenses against the suffering that is marked by such speech. Think, for example of a young man who describes himself as Atlas, holding up the world. This is the position in which he finds himself in his family of origin, accused of being the source of whatever suffering prevails. His speech is unconventional, which has resulted in various labels, including "psychotic," even though his speech is quite precise and cogent, but lodges at that odd juncture of concrete metaphor that is often called psychotic.

If, however, one allows oneself to enter into the family dialogue, one discovers the good intentions and presumptions of care that cover over the defensive moves against engaging with the speech of the identified patient. Doublings and splitting of meanings are everywhere; Paul is accused of a lack of empathy at precisely the moment when he is showing, in his own way, his recognition of the suffering of another family member. Defending what is experienced as an attack, however, family members seem unaware of his earnest efforts or the legitimacy of his pain. Rather, he is accused of caring only about himself while he sits isolated from the protective care of the family that laments his exclusion as though it were self-imposed. I find these meetings dizzying, often leaving them in need of reassurance from my co-therapist as to what has just transpired, walking away on unsteady feet, as though I had just stepped off a carnival ride.

That carnival-ride sensation also occurs at times in our engagements with one another. In some moments, our conversations are engaged and animated. At times, however, a shift suddenly occurs and I become suspect, one of *them* – those well-intentioned caregivers whose utter blindness makes them dangerous. I struggle with the me-them, insisting that there is a me guiding my speech and behaviors, but that I am also willing to think about ways in which the them in me might color or inform my speech. My willingness to struggle provides some assurance. At times, however, the stumbling is so jarring that I am thrust off balance. In one such moment, when Paul's fear had so denuded my speech of whatever meaning had been intended, I was taken aback, as though the wind had been knocked out of me. In trying to describe my experience of the moment, Paul named the Gravitron, the carnival ride in which one is thrust backward, spinning. We could both recognize that I was, for those moments, in the place where Paul spends much of his time, and how difficult it is to get one's bearings, much less think or engage with another person, from that place.

Paul's depiction of himself as Atlas seems apt, if one is willing to allow the possible meanings to accrue and resonate. Such recognition, however, requires a willingness to take one's own place on the Gravitron and to recognize how bits of meaning that are refused pile up and take their toll. Another patient recently was describing her experience of being in her family and having to fail in whatever she tried as a way to keep envy from unbalancing the system. I found myself thinking of Sisyphus and how he keeps rolling the boulder up the hill, only to have it fall once again. It occurred to me that this can seem to be the price of inclusion, that one persists in this recurrent effort on behalf of the family/culture that cannot allow one to build a path by which one might succeed. However, playing with this metaphor, I think that it is also possible that one might veer away from the injunctions of the family drama and find, at the top of the hill, a resting place or even other paths one might tread.

I told the patient that I was thinking of her use of myth, and how these myths might mark a place where one is stuck in the family, but that reflective consideration of the myth might also open up the possibility of a different ending or path. I wonder how this type of speculation might also be true of Atlas, holding up the world. His family may, in some sense, need him to stand in this position, but perhaps the world will still exist even if he lets go of his burden? From this perspective of possibility, I make this suggestion to him. My reflections bring up for me the question of how we might use myths in more creative, generative ways, beyond the recognition of an entrenched pattern. Part of what is occurring to me is the possibility of locating the myth within the constellation of the family dynamic in which it is embedded. In this way, we can see how it *becomes* universal rather than necessarily *being* universal.

Aesthetic sensibility, primary process, and metaphor

Psychoanalysis is such a dense enterprise that it is easy to become lost in accumulating knowledge rather than assimilating meanings. Pushing back against the weight of such received knowledge, I have been thinking increasingly about

Freud's rendering of libido, that primary charged energy that drives us. Through his deft, brilliant, but idiosyncratic mind and hands, that concept came to be heavily linked with sexuality over sensuality. Considering, however, my own internal workings, I find myself driven more primarily by something I would term aesthetic, profoundly embodied and affective – sensual rather than sexual.

Exploring the literature, I find that my own musings meet with those of others who have come before me. Notably, Meg Harris Williams (2005), following Donald Meltzer and Harris Williams (1988), highlights Wilfred Bion's exposition of three frames of reference: the scientific, the religious, and the aesthetic. Poring more deeply into Bion, we find him exploring this aesthetic dimension in which *passion* is a marker of the emotional truth of whatever is revealed through the senses and myth is a way of organizing these primary meanings. Through this lens, he explores the territory Freud (1900) refers to as *primary process*, and Matte-Blanco (1975) further explicates in his descriptions of *symmetrical logic*. This is the territory of the condensed and displaced, timeless and affectively laden symbolic logic of dreams.

Consistent with the notion of primary process as, precisely, *primary*, Bion (1962) outlines a theory of thinking that, in tracing the development of thought, also marks the development of the capacity to think. Presaging the current focus on reflective function as perhaps the most important process in human maturation and becoming, through Bion's lens we find an appreciation of the profound complexity of this process. Presaging Lacan's (1974–1975) *Borromean knot*, Bion highlights the importance and inevitable idiosyncrasy of perspective in meaning-making. Privileging learning over knowledge, his is a conceptualization of the human mind and being as always in motion, always moving toward or against the *catastrophic change* entailed in new learning, as we write and re-write the story of our lives. In his hands, the primal scene and Oedipal dilemma move beyond the singular myth that reveals the pattern but obscures the layering. Holding the pattern as essential to meaning-making; he helps us to accept the complexity rather than foreclosing on it, suggesting that the Oedipal myth is not so much about sexuality but rather about our tendency to *turn a blind eye* rather than facing difficult truths. Bion's notion of the *truth instinct* (Grotstein, 2004) that can guide us, if we allow it, is, I think, a recognition of the embodied nature of these primary truths, truths that form, for me, the navigational structure of individual integrity and authenticity.

There is, in psychoanalysis, a thread that follows the trail of embodied truths. Psychoanalysts such as Milner (1987), Coltart (1992), and Kristeva (1986a, 1986b) have certainly explored that territory but it remains, to my mind, insufficiently integrated into the psychoanalytic canon. Williams certainly followed that thread, as does Pistiner de Cortiña (2009) in her recognition of the value of the aesthetic domain, linking Bion's domains of myth, sense, and passion to form what she terms an *aesthetic dimension* of the mind. I would go further and suggest that what she is locating as an aspect of mind is more fundamental. From my perspective, this aesthetic sensibility is actually closer to what Freud was pointing to in his depictions of libido, which originally were profoundly sensual rather than more narrowly sexual. This domain would seem to be the source of what psychoanalysts refer to as unconscious or preconscious experience, *primary* process.

As psychoanalysts, we say we believe in the unconscious. We *theorize* about it, we *recognize* its workings in our patients, but our surprise when we encounter it shows the extent of our *dis*belief. For example, in a recent seminar on dreams and field theory, my students and I were deep into the investigation of dreams, beginning first with Freud's (1900) own explorations and insights, as he discusses them in Chapter 7 of *The Interpretation of Dreams*. During the second evening, a student highlighted a concept from Green (1999) that had been used in one of the texts. I was having trouble understanding the concept of *negative hallucination* within the context of this particular text. A student very simply described it, saying that "it is like when this pen is here but you do not see it." That made sense as it stood, but the author of the text was saying that, developmentally, the negative hallucination was necessary for representation to occur. This idea seemed to me to be quite similar to Winnicott's (1971) idea that one must be able to make the thing re-appear in order to be able to represent it. For whatever reason, I seemed to be too stuck in rational logic to be able to access the more symmetrical logic through which whatever we might make re-appear, we must also be able to make *dis*-appear. In an attempt to resolve the questions that continued to elude me, we went back to the text we had been reading.

The idea offered by Perelberg (2016) seemed to be that the mother's arms structure an experience such that in her absence something can be represented to fill the gap. "The capacity for the negative hallucination of the mother lies at the origins of representation; it is against the background of negativity that future representations of the object are inscribed. This is the role of the negative in its structuring function" (p. 1575). I could only make sense of this statement in relation to notions of the internalization of the absent object that enables the individual to sustain contact and endure the absence. From that frame of reference, my student's explanation made no sense. She found a later paper from Green where he was using this concept, but the negative hallucination was being linked to other ideas in ways that, for me, merely further muddied the waters.

We continued to explore the various texts we had read for that day. I had the sense that this concept of the negative hallucination had not been offered sufficiently clearly to the uninformed reader to be able to follow Perelberg's arguments. I was then left with a lovely poetry that had carried me along sufficiently to have derived a sense of felt-value and to have assigned the text, even though my conscious mind could not fully comprehend important aspects of it.

The following morning, I looked up this concept on the Internet and found a very clear and concise description that was precisely what the student had originally offered. I sent the students an email with the definition, along with the further noted fact that the idea had originated in Freud (Breuer & Freud, 1893–1895) but had been expanded by Green (1999). I then pointed out to them how mag-nificently my unconscious mind had manifested the concept that my conscious mind had refused to grasp, giving examples of how I had muddied the water by insisting on exploring the unclear text rather than the student's clear description. I also noted how I had further, again unconsciously, illustrated the concept by (seemingly randomly) talking about how I sometimes confuse myself when I see a familiar face but then wonder if it is not actually the person I know but rather only someone who looks like them. In the face of the refusal of meaning, enact-ments were everywhere.

At that evening's seminar, I discussed with the students the dilemma they had been in. I mentioned how easy it had been for me to look up the concept. They each had a laptop or other device in front of them, and yet no one had checked. I told them that I suspected that, in the reverse situation, if the student had been wrong, someone would have Googled the concept to clarify. I said that this should be a lesson to us, inviting us to advocate more actively for a position that seems right to us, so that we can each continue to look at a complicated issue from various sides rather than closing down the conversation by deferring to someone else's authority.

It seemed to me that in our earnest efforts to understand this complicated issue of dreams from various perspectives – including the field theories that insist that we extend our scope beyond the dream itself to the ways in which the uncon-scious meanings that speak from within the dream also speak in myriad ways – we were able to appreciate something about the psychoanalytic process *because we were watching ourselves living it*. This incident served as a reminder that we each possess an unconscious and that it is, indeed, unconscious and yet we can catch glimpses of whatever is missing from precisely the types of slips, symptoms, and enactments that psychoanalysis has illuminated.

During that same period of time, I had been reading Pistiner de Cortiña's (2009) work on the aesthetic dimension of the mind because of my own suspicion that the aesthetic is not just a dimension of the mind but rather points to something more profound, the underlying substrate of what is termed the primary process. Pistiner de Cortiña invokes Bion's (1977) extensions into sense, myth, and passion to point to the ways in which the unconscious registers and lodges meanings. I had been suspecting that this formula affords a better understanding of libido itself – the primary motivating force that became skewed toward the sexual in ways that mask and trivialize its more diverse meanings and profound essence. Is not the libido, rather, the most primary message from the unconscious, the term marking the ways in which Matte-Blanco's (1975) unconscious logic both calls to us and eludes us, formulating itself so that the conscious mind might grasp the meanings and heed the call?

Were not all of my acting-outs within the seminar also ways of trying to express and expose a concept my conscious mind refused to grasp? In this way, was I not, paradoxically, trying to do what I value most – invite my students to learn from their own experience and thereby to constitute themselves as knowers, subjects in their own right, rather than using me to subvert their own becoming by placing me – illegitimately – in the place of the primary knower?

Limit, the maternal, and subjectification

There is a part of us that yearns for some authority in whose mind and arms we can rest, and yet, no one can fully know the heart, soul, and mind of another. Growth requires the capacity to encounter and tolerate limits so that we can constitute ourselves as separate yet interrelated beings. In these efforts, we must all, to some extent, grapple with maternal failures that leave fragments of meanings undigested and seemingly off-limits, dangerous, or incomprehensible.

From Bion's (1977) perspective, maternal failures leave in the infant the bits and fragment that remain as beta elements – undigested and undigestible. It remains for these elements to emerge in the presence of empathic interest and curiosity so that they can be felt, recognized, and thought about. Until that point, they remain the ever-present companions that destroy any efforts toward development, marking such attempts as false because the bombardment does not cease but rather lies perpetually in wait to dislodge us and expose the lie. The undigested fact that can be recognized may be uncomfortable or even awful, but its recognition springs the trap and makes it possible to take steps that have grounding to them. We become real. This seems to be the realm of Lacan's (1978) *objet petit a*, that points to the reckoning with truth that makes it possible to constitute ourselves as a legitimate subject – one unique voice in the conversation.

From that place, what is unique in us can come forward in ways that invite our interest and curiosity. We can better tolerate the unknown that emerges and play with it, in the service of the interrelated efforts of art-making and meaning-making. Such a stance is essential for all those who attempt to provide care for vulnerable individuals. Without sufficient respect for the legitimacy of precisely the otherness of the other, attempts at containment can become an impossible prison, foreclosing growth rather than facilitating it. Whatever our hopes and beliefs, we can only serve the other in relation to his or her desire. For example, I worked with a young man who considered himself to be a "mad" painter. His painting took place during frenzied periods in the wee hours of the night and then closed down. His painting instructor took the position that this young man was actually a gifted artist, but the young man's relationship with himself and his creativity was such that he did not believe that he could sustain his life and also his art. At that juncture, he turned away from both art-making and also the meaning-making he was working at in his psychoanalytic treatment. That moment has stayed with me over the years, mirroring other artist's fears and investments in a certain price to be paid for the gift of creation.

As someone whose art sprang from my distress, I can well understand that pivotal moment when, distress attenuated, one has lost the source of one's inspiration.

However, I also know that it is possible to find new, untapped resources within oneself through which to continue one's creative efforts. Psychoanalysis and other insight-oriented therapies do not necessarily work toward the type of "normalization" at times feared by creative individuals. Rather, there is an appreciation in theorists as diverse as Winnicott and Lacan of the importance of the consulting room in providing a space where an individual subject can emerge in all their uniqueness.

> If the child hidden within each grown adult is the cause of his mental suffering, this child is also the source of art and of the poetry of life. On his continuing existence rests the ever-present promise of a fresh perception of the world, the revelation of unsuspected mystery in the everyday scene, the maintenance of a personal and private folly to offset the deadening specter of "normative normality" which adulthood might bring. It is the task of each of us to know how to keep in touch with the magical and narcissistic child within, so that he may not be stifled. To see this exchange take place with the patient in analysis is a moving experience; to see it fail, a tragedy.
>
> (McDougall, 1980, p. 18)

Creation and destruction: the use of an object

Milner (1987) notes that when reality has intruded too harshly, too soon, self-development – and the use of symbols for meaning-making – is impeded. For such individuals, the illusion of symbiotic oneness with the analyst provides a vehicle through which the self can be discovered. In relation to this type of developmental process, Milner notes that:

> It seemed as if it was only by being able, again and again, to experience the illusion that I was part of himself, fused with the goodness that he could conceive of internally, that he became able to tolerate a goodness that was not his own creation and to allow me goodness independently.
>
> (p. 193)

Milner's focus seems to be in line with Winnicott's (1971) *use of the object*, in which he marks the importance of the object's ability to withstand attacks sufficiently to remain available. Because the goodness in the other can survive, there is the presumption of goodness in oneself – in spite of the bad – that can still be recognized. It is only in a world in which there can be destruction that there can be creation.

> The basic identifications which make it possible to find new objects, to find the familiar in the unfamiliar, require an ability to tolerate a temporary loss of sense of self, a temporary giving up of the discriminating ego

which stands apart and tries to see things objectively and rationally and without emotional coloring.

(Milner, p. 189)

Just as psychoanalysis attempts to make the unconscious conscious, to give words to ephemeral, yet deeply felt, experience, so too "the artist wishes to cast his private experiences in such form that they will be incorporated in the social world of art and thus lessen the discrepancy" (Milner, pp. 190–191). This type of interchange, however, requires sufficient ego integrity that one can survive encounters with another being or idea. For Winnicott (1968), this possibility depends on the possibility of playing.

> *Psychotherapy takes place in the overlap of two areas of playing, that of the patient and that of the therapist. Psychotherapy has to do with two people playing together. The corollary of this is that where playing is not possible then the work done by the therapist is directed towards bringing the patient from a state of not being able to play into a state of being able to play.*

(p. 591, italics in original)

Creative efforts necessarily require destruction of whatever has come before in order to move forward, to take the project further toward the goal that has not even truly been imagined. Rather, we encounter the lack, and try to work with it to transform it, to soften the edges or embolden the outlines, working toward the integrity of the project as it emerges. This is the process described by artists of all sorts, to eliminate the chaff and allow the scene to unfold and the characters to speak for themselves. Ehrenzweig (1967) describes this process in relation to a *hidden order* in the unconscious that is more accessible through creative efforts than through rational logic. Within the consulting room, Coltart (1992), following both Freud and Bion, suggests that it is faith that enables us to wait for the pattern to emerge, rather than imposing meaning in ways that obstruct the potential becoming of that individual.

Langer (1953) goes further, driving back toward the essential link between feeling, form, and aesthetic sensibilities that underlies the symbolic meanings apprehended through the nonverbal channels. That link is also apparent in the term *faith*, as used by Coltart, which recognizes something ineffable and potentially transformative the drives the human spirit.

Fromm (1950) recognizes this urge toward the transcendent as a fundamental human need, what Bion (1977) terms the *aesthetic dimension* of experience; what I call an *aesthetic sensibility*. If we think of the aesthetic in the terms offered by Gadamer (1975), as something that disrupts and thereby reveals cultural limits and expectations, then we are in the territory of an experience of truth that moves beyond the particular into the universal. This is also the territory of Bion's (1977) *truth instinct*, the suggestion that there is something in us that can move toward either truth or evasion. Human development requires a frame within which we can come into finer attunement with an internal sense of truth and integrity, a moral authority that is authorized, not by an external being, but rather an internal sensibility.

Truth, meaning, and the outer reaches of human sensibilities

Gadamer's (1975) attempts to define and historicize ideas about the aesthetic in relation to his ideas about truth and method are very much in line with Bion's (1977) ideas about a passion that marks something of essential importance but also can drive us utterly astray. My experience is that those we call psychotic are often mystics who have lost their way. In current times, when we are wary of spirituality and have largely lost track of the structures through which we might meet our mystics with reverence, we tend to drive those seeking truth into the wilderness of the psychiatric establishment. The answers to be found in that realm have little to do with truth-seeking – moving, rather, into the realm of problem solving. It *matters* whether we see human suffering as an integral part of living, to be understood, worked with, and worked through, or whether we see such suffering as a mark of aberration to be reduced or eliminated. These are fundamentally different values that orient our efforts in markedly different directions.

If we are to locate the plight of such sufferers in relation to an abject marginalization, then the challenge becomes to try to create the conditions for engagement between two individuals. That brings us to Winnicott (1971), for whom *play* forms the bedrock, not only for interpersonal engagement, but also for the universe of subjective, creative, and aesthetic experience. This is also the domain of Lacan's (1977a, 1977b) *Imaginary*, designated as the realm in which one person's constructions coexist with those of others. For Lacan, the *Symbolic*, the realm of laws and language, binds us together but also, less explored in his writings, so too does the *Real*. As the realm of what is left out, left over, left unexplained, the numinous would seem to inhabit the realm of the Real. Linking these theories and theoreticians together, we see the problem they are faced with, that we do indeed have experiences that point us toward what may arise out of self-other experience but also transcend and transform it. In that way, psychoanalysis functions best when it provides a model of development, such as that offered by Loewald (1978a), who, similar to Bion's (1977) transformation of Klein's theories, shifts away from Freud's presumptions regarding a linear path of development toward one that is recursive, replenished through the unconscious in ways that allow a new synthesis, based, I would contend, on aesthetic, feeling-based principles rather than on rational logic.

We find theorizing on these issues in literature that looks at spiritual experience, as in Jones (2002), who locates the realm of aesthetic or religious ecstatic experience in relation to a sense of time that is transformed, in Loewald's words, "by the timelessness of the unconscious or primary process" (1978b, p. 67), through which familiar forms and patterns of experience resonate in ways that are profound and experience-near. The encounter with such primary truths can be both tantalizing and terrifying, making it important to be able to find solid ground on which to stand. The consulting room can provide that type of containment, within which the patterns can be recognized and, along with them, emergent symbols that bring us into the realm of myth and metaphor. Symbols "enable us to play with aspects of experience that are not accessible to conscious thought, including whatever might be too terrifying if it were to be perceived as too 'real'" (Charles, 2005, p. 487), but we can only play with symbols if there is sufficient containment within the social surround (Charles, forthcoming).

Bollas' (1987) notion of the *transformative object* presumes a legitimate, developmental move toward transformation through another being that is modeled on the parent/child relationship. In contrast, Lacan's (1977b) concern over the possibility of becoming lost in relation to another pushes his stance away from this dangerous intermingling. His caution is well taken: we are always in danger of becoming *lost* in another rather than *finding ourselves* through the relationship with another. We cannot develop, we cannot *become* without an immersion in the experience of being, but we need respectful encounters with other, separate, sentient beings in order to find our way. As Loewald, Bion, and Winnicott each stress in their own ways, knowing-about is not the same as knowing, and true development proceeds through an integration of the mind and body, thought and feeling, secondary and primary experience; in Matte-Blanco's (1975) terms, conscious and unconscious logics.

This distinction between knowing for oneself versus knowing-about seems inherent in Buber's (1970) distinction between an I-it and an I-you relationship, echoing the distinction made previously between authority-driven therapy models versus person-centered approaches. Notably, that intensely authentic quality of engagement and relatedness is also likely fundamental to an experience of the numinous or sacred (Jones, 2002). This creative area of transitional space has been described by Kristeva (1986c) in terms of the *chora*, the underlying rhythmic, energic patterning of experience upon which our coming-into-being rests. She contrasts a *logic of identification* that locates itself within the dominant, more rational discourse of society, with a *dynamic of signs* that refuses linear temporality in favor of an aesthetic, embodied, spiritual discourse that calls to us more directly. Neuropsychological studies affirm the essential organizing structure of aesthetic sensibilities, suggesting "that humans have an intuitive feel for the complexity of self-similar patterns, showing evidence for the aesthetic preferences for fractal-like auditory and visual patterns" (Mirón, 2019, p. 49).

Language provides a fundamental bond between people but is also at odds with other ways of making meaning that are driven by affect or, in Kristeva's words "the infinitesimal significations with the relationships with the nature of their own bodies" (1986a, p. 199). Working with those who have been pushed aside from consensual discourse demand that we continually re-orient ourselves in line with our own sensibilities, as best we can locate and understand them. The allegiance to that type of internal truth marks a crucial ethical injunction that we also see in Bion and Lacan, who place a personal ethics, Bion's *truth instinct* (Grotstein, 2004; originally described in terms of *passion* in Bion, 1977) or Lacan's (1992) *desire of the subject*, at the heart of profound intrapsychic development.

In this way, Kristeva (1982, 1986b) traces a path of potential development that can only come in an embodied form, not through the pillars of received knowledge but rather through the personal feelings that arise from facing limit. This leads, she suggests,

> to the active research, still rare, undoubtedly hesitant but always dissident, being carried out by women in the human sciences; particularly those attempts, in the wake of contemporary art, to break the code, to shatter language, to find a discourse closer to the body and emotions, to the unnameable repressed by the social contract.
>
> (1986b, p. 200)

In this way, Kristeva invites us to break through the constrictions of the social world that can become a "sacrificial contract" (p. 200) in which our very soul is likely at stake. Denying the profundity of these choices, for the clinician, threatens to put at stake the very being of the other, particularly those who have been marginalized and deemed incompetent through a perhaps well-intentioned but inevitably deadly *epistemic injustice* (Fricker, 2007) that denies the validity of the subject himself or herself, marginalizing the person as primary knower of their own experience.

In addressing the more primary, affective functions of language, Kristeva's position is similar to that of Lacan (1977b), when he writes, "the function of language is not to inform but to evoke" (p. 86). Language poses a particular problem in that it speaks and hides in relation to our ambivalent desire to know and to be known. And yet, inevitably, we reveal ourselves: "the symptom *is* metaphor whether one likes it or not, as desire *is* metonymy" (Lacan, 1977c, p. 175, italics in original).

And yet, in the search for meaning – and for safety – we also must seek answers from without in order to anchor and organize our experience. Campbell (1988) notes that the position of the shaman, whose wisdom comes from direct experience, marks the allure and aversion to direct knowledge. For Campbell, the shaman is the character who uses externally sanctioned authority to invite recognition of internal truths, in that way serving a similar function to that of the psychoanalyst, and also the mystic and the psychotic. Those who speak from beyond consensual knowledge are both desired and feared, but also potentially form a bridge between internal and external truths in relation to one's own authenticity.

Human development depends upon the external vantage point that helps to contain and to organize our experience, but always in relation to our emergent capacity to make our own meanings in line with an internal sense of truth. That truth is always based on the internal, embodied, aesthetic experience that anchors us in a truth that can be expanded upon as we learn more about self-in-relation-to-other but cannot be essentially countermanded by any other. This is the realm of T. S. Eliot's (1934) old stones that need deciphering. Psychoanalysis provides a means for engaging in a process whereby one's old stones might be deciphered as part of a developmental process that Gadamer (1975) would term a *transformation into the true*.

References

Bion, W. R. (1962). A theory of thinking. *International Journal of Psycho-Analysis*, *43*(4–5), 306–310.

Bion, W. R. (1977). *Seven servants*. London: Heinemann.

Bollas, C. (1987). *The shadow of the object*. New York: Columbia University Press.

Breuer, J., & Freud, S. (1893–1895). Studies on hysteria. In *Standard edition* (Vol. 2). London: Hogarth Press, 1971.

Buber, M. (1970). *I and thou* (W. Kaufman, Trans.). New York: Scribner's.

Campbell, J. (1988). *The power of myth*. New York: Viking Press.

Charles, M. (2005). Patterns: Basic units of emotional memory. *Psychoanalytic Inquiry*, *25*(4), 484–505.

Charles, M. (2010a). Epiphany: The poet's Art, the analyst's instrument. Formal structure as a vehicle for the expression of primary experience. *Psychoanalytic Review*, *97*, 451–467.

Charles, M. (2010b). When cultures collide: Myth, meaning, and configural space. *Modern Psychoanalysis*, *34*, 26–47.

Charles, M. (2015). *Psychoanalysis and literature: The stories we live*. Lanham, MD: Rowman & Littlefield.

Charles, M. (forthcoming). Mysticism and madness: A matter of perspective? In I. Lambrecht & A. Lavis (Eds.), *Culture and psychosis*. Routledge. ISPS Book Series.

Charles, M., & Telis, K. (2014). Pattern as inspiration and mode of communication in the works of Van Gogh. In M. G. Fromm (Ed.), *A spirit that impels: Play, creativity, and psychoanalysis* (pp. 95–121). London: Karnac Books.

Coltart, N. (1992). *Slouching towards Bethlehem*. New York: Guilford Press.

Ehrenzweig, A. (1967). *The hidden order of art: A study in the psychology of artistic imagination*. London: Weidenfeld and Nicolson.

Eliot, T. S. (1934). Four quartets. In *Collected poems: 1909–1962* (pp. 175–209). New York: Harcourt, Brace and World.

Freud, S. (1900/1971). The interpretation of dreams. In *Standard edition* (Vol. 4–5). London: Hogarth Press.

Fricker, M. (2007). *Epistemic injustice: Power and the ethics of knowing*. Oxford: Oxford University Press.

Fromm, E. (1950). *Psychoanalysis and religion*. New Haven: Yale University Press.

Gadamer, H.-G. (1975). *Truth and method*. New York: Continuum.

Gallese, V. (2009). Mirror neurons, embodied simulation, and the neural basis of social identification. *Psychoanalytic Dialogues*, *19*, 519–536.

Green, A. (1972). *On private madness*. Madison, WI: International Universities Press.

Green, A. (1999). *The work of the negative*. London: Free Association Books.

Grotstein, J. S. (2004). The seventh servant: The implications of a truth drive in Bion's theory of 'O'. *International Journal of Psychoanalysis, 85*, 1081–1101.

Jones, J. W. (2002). The experience of the holy: A relational psychoanalytic analysis. *Pastoral Psychology, 50*(3), 153–164.

Kristeva, J. (1982). *Powers of horror: An essay on abjection* (L. S. Roudiez, Trans.). New York: Columbia University Press.

Kristeva, J. (1986a). Stabat mater. In T. Moi (Ed.), *The Kristeva reader* (L. S. Roudiez & S. Hand, Trans., pp. 160–186). New York: Columbia University Press.

Kristeva, J. (1986b). Women's time. In T. Moi (Ed.), *The Kristeva reader* (L. S. Roudiez & S. Hand, Trans., pp. 187–213). New York: Columbia University Press.

Kristeva, J. (1986c). Revolution in poetic language. In T. Moi (Ed.), *The Kristeva reader* (L. S. Roudiez & S. Hand, Trans., pp. 89–136). New York: Columbia University Press.

Lacan, J. (1974–1975). *Seminar XII: RSI* (C. Gallagher, Trans.). www.lacaninireland.com/web/published-works/seminars.

Lacan, J. (1977a). The subversion of the subject and the dialectic of desire in the Freudian unconscious. In A. Sheridan (Trans.), *Écrits* (pp. 292–325). New York: W. W. Norton & Company.

Lacan, J. (1977b). The function and field of speech and language in psychoanalysis. In A. Sheridan (Trans.), *Écrits* (pp. 30–113). New York: W. W. Norton & Company.

Lacan, J. (1977c). The agency of the letter in the unconscious or reason since Freud. In A. Sheridan (Trans.), *Écrits* (pp. 146–178). New York: W. W. Norton & Company.

Lacan, J. (1978). *The four fundamentals of psychoanalysis* (J.-A. Miller, Ed., A. Sheridan, Trans.). New York: W. W. Norton & Company.

Lacan, J. (1992). *The ethics of psychoanalysis* (J.-A. Miller, Ed., D. Porter, Trans.). New York: W. W. Norton & Company.

Langer, S. K. (1953). *Feeling and form: A theory of art developed from philosophy in a new key*. New York: Scribner's.

Levinas, E. (1999). *Alterity and transcendence* (M. B. Smith, Trans.). New York: Columbia University Press.

Loewald, H. (1978a). Primary process, secondary process, and language. In *Papers on Psychoanalysis* (pp. 178–206). New Haven: Yale University Press, 1980.

Loewald, H. (1978b). *Psychoanalysis and the history of the individual*. New Haven, CT: Yale University Press.

Matte-Blanco, I. (1975). *The unconscious as infinite sets: An essay in bi-logic*. London: Duckworth.

McDougall, J. (1980). *Plea for a measure of abnormality*. New York: International Universities Press.

Meltzer, D., & Harris Williams, M. (1988). *The apprehension of beauty*. Old Ballechin, Scotland: Clunie Press.

Milner, M. (1987). *The suppressed madness of sane men: Forty-four years of exploring psychoanalysis*. London: Tavistock.

Mirón, M. (2019). *Metapsychology and complexity: Implications for psychoanalysis*. Masters Thesis. Universidad de Monterrey, Monterrey.

Perelberg, R. J. (2016). Negative hallucinations, dreams and hallucinations: The framing structure and its representation in the analytic setting. *International Journal of Psychoanalysis, 97*, 1575–1590.

Pistiner de Cortiña, L. (2009). *The aesthetic dimension of the mind: Variations on a theme of Bion.* London: Karnac Books.

Seikkula, J., Aaltonen, J., Alakare, B., Haarakangas, K., Keränen, J., & Lehtinen, K. (2006). Five-year experience of first-episode nonaffective psychosis in open-dialogue approach: Treatment principles, follow-up outcomes, and two case studies. *Psychotherapy Research, 16*(2), 214–228.

Suomi, S. J. (2011). Risk, resilience, and gene-environment interplay in primates. *Journal of the Canadian Academy of Child and Adolescent Psychiatry, 20*(4), 289–297.

Thalbourne, M. A., Bartemucci, L., Delin, P. S., Fox, B., & Nofi, O. (1997). Transliminality: Its nature and correlates. *Journal of the American Society for Psychical Research, 91*, 305–331.

Thalbourne, M. A., & Delin, P. S. (1999). Transliminality: Its relation to dream life, religiosity, and mystical experience. *International Journal for the Psychology of Religion, 9*(1), 45–61.

Vanheule, S. (2011). *The subject of psychosis: A Lacanian perspective.* London: Palgrave Macmillan.

Williams, M. H. (2005). The three vertices: Science, art and religion. *British Journal of Psychotherapy, 21*(3), 429–441.

Winnicott, D. W. (1968). Playing: Its theoretical status in the clinical situation. *International Journal of Psycho-Analysis, 49*, 591–599.

Winnicott, D. W. (1971). *Playing and reality.* London: Routledge.

Chapter 10

Soul is crying

Michael Eigen

ABSTRACT: This chapter touches upon three individuals who suffered psychotic breakdowns and underwent hospitalizations with medication regimes. Two discovered transformational possibilities in severed and shattered states. The third was helped to cope with a semi-reduced lifestyle compared to what he once envisioned but found creative and relational satisfaction. All became hospital free and two medication free. The author brings together common themes, images, and ideas growing out of raw experience of breakdown, with awareness that selections are partial and suggestive.

KEYWORDS: psychosis, breakdown, psychoanalysis, Winnicott, Bion

So many conflicting, paradoxical views are expressed about psychosis. For some, madness can be a gateway to transcendent vision. For others, madness connotes a deep sense of rejection and disability. There are many points in between and mixes that exceed categories. If I've learned anything, it's to stay open to differences and surprise. Wilfred Bion quipped that life is filled with surprises, most of them bad. Too often one hears of something going well, then tragedy hits. Bion (1970) often writes of a good feeling state going bad while Winnicott (1965) often covers the opposite ground, movements from bad feeling states to better (Eigen, 2002, 2004). A kind of double rhythm that when working well can lead to growth, a life rhythm one learns to work with. Good to bad, bad to good: it takes making room for, waiting out, working with.

The work reported here implicitly revolves around making room for the double rhythm of bad and good states reversing, transforming into each other, moving beyond themselves, a kind of rhythm of faith that all is not bad, that a good seed is worth planting and growing. If there are times the good does not survive the bad, there are also times in this primal rhythm when the good does survive and promises something further. A profoundly worthwhile kernel, however infinitesimal, keeps opening possibilities of life.

Alma

We begin with tears, some of them seen, some unseen, heard soundlessly within. Alma comes in one day saying, "Alma is crying. Alma is crying."

It was almost as if Alma was a little girl watching her mother helpless in tears, a scene she often witnessed in childhood. Her mother convulsed in tears, doubled over on the floor or hiding in bed. She does not remember how young she was when her mother's tears began telling her, "You should never have been born." At first, she thought she heard her mother actually speaking to her, but no, her mother remained in wordless agony, communicating through crying sounds. The translation into words came through the tears themselves, as if they could speak – in fact, for Alma, they did speak. They accused her of being the cause of her mother's pain. And often her own mind translated this into being her mother's pain, a formulation that coagulated into the words, "I am my mother's pain." A stubborn, persistent identity feeling that informed her life.

Sometimes when these words came out, I might wonder aloud, "Is your mother your pain, too?" A pain passed on through generations, perhaps related to the pain of life? How does the pain of life get funneled through ego, self, personality, so that I and/or you become the cause of pain? "The" cause or "a" cause? The pain of life gets funneled into causal thinking, "I" and "you" being two of the main causal characters (Eigen, 2005).

In the small field of family dynamics, the pain of life, among other things, becomes the pain mother and child inflict on each other. Pain is part of the interactive field with oneself and others. But how we view it, interpret it, what kind of affective framework builds around it, varies. Interpretations can add to or modulate the pain they address. Persecutory voices can be horrifying interpretations of the pain of life.

Alma and I have been working together over eight years. She had several hospital stays before we began. I am aware we are working millimeters over rivers of intense fragility, although she herself more often feels under or in rather than over. Nevertheless, so far she is surviving herself and some of the enormous strength of persecutory feelings has slowly become part of strength she can use for herself. Is it an odd thought to imagine some of the force of self-attack is a kind of reservoir holding strength waiting for us to learn how to use?

There came a time I could ask, "Is it really you crying? Alma, is it really you?"

Could one tell if she had become her mother crying? Who was crying for whom? Did it matter whose pain was being expressed? Could one tell? For years it could as easily been her mother crying as her and the accusing voices her mother's tears transformed to.

At the moment I am touching on now Alma said, "Yes, it's me, really me, at least a little. There is a little of me here."

For the moment, it was not simply feeling blamed for being alive or blaming the other for blaming her. At the moment, the blame of the voice diminished and a cry closer to the heart of existence, the pain of life could be felt and shared. In a way her saying, "Alma is crying. Alma is crying," was a call asking for response, a shared moment and it was my job to honor it. Amidst the debris of awfulness was a cry of existence seeking recognition, caring, sharing. We had reached a threshold where the strength of fragility could be respected and not simply turned against itself.

In such moments, a little is a lot. How devastating it was that for years of her life, she lived at the edge of being demolished by negative voices and fear of them. Voices not only telling her bad things about herself but also threatening punishments that were terrifying, unbearable. There are so many ways to live at the edge of annihilation, in this case psychic annihilation, dread of one's being. And now, at least, there was a little clearing, a little bit of life-feeling she could say yes to, a bit of positive self-recognition, self-caring, self-kindness. A new current was forming and she could feel and share it. We could acknowledge it together.

"Alma is crying" was Alma's way of making contact with herself in face of and in spite of bad voices and accusations. It took quite some perseverance and persistence to reach this point. I'm tempted to say that it took a modicum of unconscious faith, a refusal to believe she was all bad even though time and again the voices insisted that she was. Bad and unredeemable. I think of the biblical cry, "Save me, O Lord!" Indeed, save me from myself. Save me from the endless pain of my life. Save me from my life so that I may give life.

The turning point was slow coming but had its own cumulative strength, and Alma began wondering where she could make use of the life she was discovering. To be a helper for people with difficulties like hers was a possible path that took hold and at this writing she is well on her way to exploring ways to do this. To help others with difficulties one deals with and finds openings through is a way to help oneself by helping others and helping others by helping oneself.

Philip

Philip grew up feeling that big things were expected of him. He played games with other children but also spent a lot of time alone. He felt pain in both situations – and pleasures, too. It was difficult to say which comforted him more, as if he needed cushioning from both. Perhaps it was simply the intensity of being that was difficult, the baffling intensity of being alive. Many years later, he found himself wondering whether his difficulty arose from or was compounded by the fact that no one ever taught him what to do with the intensity of life. It was never mentioned, not at home or in school. One went from activity to activity, rush and quiet but somehow the raw fact of what life felt like was not part of education. The very fact of being and what it felt like escaped notice and talk.

Later he found hints of it in poetry and thought there must be some link between his name, Philip, and *phil*osophy. But what could "lip" mean? Kissing? Or somehow associated with anger – "Don't give me any lip, youngster." "Bite your lip" seemed associated with something bad inside which mustn't come out. Don't say it. It must stay hidden within, whatever it was. The therapy invitation to "say whatever is in you" seemed the opposite of his home and education, where you had to be very careful to keep a lot to yourself. It was not clear for some time whether therapy was a relief or another kind of threat – or both.

It would take years to explore its possibilities and limitations. As he would say a bit past the beginning, "I still don't know whether it's a good idea for me to be doing this, but some scary awful thing seems a little less heavy." In time, we would be able to partly translate this to mean his inner life was beginning to feel a tiny bit less menacing, although threat and menace and punishment were never too far away.

The menace of intensity was often dismissed with words like, "Oh, Philip, he is so sensitive." He was also considered smart, with much expected. He tested exceptionally high in school and while he might often see things other students didn't, he had an inner sense that he could not keep up, that he lagged behind in something basic that eluded him. He could not find the words for it, but knew something was missing, wrong, deficient.

No one expected him to be hospitalized in his second year of college, at least so it seemed. When he came out and returned to school with the help of his first therapist he, amazingly (his feeling), discovered others in school who went through something similar, a kind of underground of sensitive intelligentsia that shared breakdown and hospital. He would have another hospital stay in transition into his 20s, but somewhere in the morass felt appreciation that he was surviving and had not perished in illness and suicide, which was all too real. Whatever was wrong, he remained, at least intermittently, in contact with something he valued, hard to say what, something to do with the preciousness of being. Something – again hard say what it was – a sense of inestimable value of seeing it through.

Much later in therapy, we could speak of "outlasting some of the bad states." Not just waiting them out, although that was part of it – but a developing sense that more could happen, part of an unconscious faith that all this is worth it. It was moving that such a sense could be there as part of an underpinning while so much had to be gone through. Is a sense of going through too much a permanent part of what being alive feels like? Is that part of our predicament we need to assimilate, make room for, live with?

It took a good many years for Philip to one day begin to say, "I don't think I can break down anymore. I don't mean breakdowns of everyday life, but hospital breakdowns. Something is shifting. It's not mainly that I'm stronger. I don't think strength is the main factor. You can be strong one day and find yourself hospitalized the next. It's more like something grew – in a way, got bigger. Not just that I can take more, although that's important. You talk about "making room." I think something like that happened, is happening. More room for me, what's in me, the wood critters, scary presences, wounds, voids. Not that I can't be done in by myself. One can't take the threat of oneself for granted. But there is more and the more has a say too. You can count on going further if you stick it out."

"It's amazing, isn't it?" I interjected, a kind of Greek chorus. "Having a psyche, being a psychical being. Not being done in by oneself. Or being done in by oneself and surviving a little at a time. Surviving being done in a little better and better still. It doesn't stop, does it?"

I wonder if I was thinking of Samuel Beckett's writing of "failing better," but I became aware Philip had taken the ball and was moving along. He had moved back to a discordance he felt since childhood. Philip:

I don't know when I began to feel more and more strongly I could not keep up with myself. The self that went so quickly and saw so much and the self that could do so little. The self that fell apart and the self that drove it. The mind that keeps pedaling faster and faster, and the mind that cannot move, stuck in speed and paralysis. The whole system needed time off from itself. Maybe the hospital was a way of getting time off – but not really. What I'm doing now works better, but there's a long way to go. There's always a long way to go. And yet – here I am talking with you, to you – or with myself to myself. Dipping in, sharing.

I don't know who I was supposed to be, but whatever, whoever it was, I didn't get there. A famous this, a great that – CEO, statesman, author, artist – someone to look up to, applaud. I think of a show with the words "lords of the universe." So many failed gods – and perhaps super-gods as well. The ancient Greeks pointed to a fatal flaw, pride, blinded by greatness. Now I see rats on a treadmill, but that's only a little part of it. We've talked about the transmission of grandiose expectations and the me that got left out, the me that couldn't move. It's exhausting to have a mind, a psyche.

I will tell you a secret. What a relief it is to go to school five days a week and teach a class. No, not famous. No Big Deal. Just a relief to be a person doing something worth doing. Sometimes touching someone in a way that makes a difference, even a little difference. There I am in front of a class, someone who has gone through the unbelievable – and the unbelievable never stops. There I am, someone sharing experience, sharing thought. Hoping against hope that something good happens, can happen. I can't tell you how lucky I feel to be just me, not a surplus version.

This past week, I've been assigning Elizabethan poems and going over them in class. I was struck by a contrast between images of city and pastoral life, busyness and ease, frenzy and calm. As the students and I were talking, I found myself applying the poems to my own turmoil and rest. Not exactly speed and paralysis but hyper and calm, a clearing and a jumble. My mind jumped to the words "getting and spending we lay waste our powers." What powers was the poet speaking of? Certainly not the power my injured mind imagined.

You speak of creative waiting, going through, outlasting, letting something else happen. How I had to endure inner accusations of being a disappointment to myself. I found my way to being a high school teacher, something I liked and could do. And accusations threatened to derail me. What does one do with the sense of disappointment? Can one outlast being a disappointment to oneself?

I'll tell you another secret, a secret we share between us. You encouraged me to open the Door of Disappointment and walk into the ominous room. You held my hand and then the door shut and I was all alone, deeper into the disappointment with myself. Terrified when walls of my personality began to close. I waited to be crushed by them. But as they got closer, I touched one and it opened like a curtain, then another curtain and another. There seemed to be no end to what could close and open in such mysterious ways. I was dumbfounded. Dumb and found. Disappointment-expectation, twins throughout a lifetime, opening-closing experience.

I think I only have room for one more secret today. And as I say that, I realize the secret is more between me and me than me and you. My own secret and discovery. I noticed Rochelle looking at me in the lunchroom and the hall and she made the first move, coming over and speaking with me. How would I spoil it? But that was just the point – learning there's life beyond spoiling. We spoil life millions of times and move with and past the spoiling. We learn to tolerate and work with disappointment, disappointing each other, disappointing ourselves.

Is this the biggest miracle of all – that disappointment can be humanizing? Going through disappointment with myself made me more human? Rochelle and I were semi-newish teachers in the school and gravitated toward each other, but she did most of the beginning work. I think she felt my humanness growing or maybe she felt we could be human together. Whatever it was, little by little, we grew together. What I feared was a reduced life turned out to make life possible.

Rochelle, too, has her story. She is not a hospital survivor, but she is an abuse survivor. She never was hospitalized, and I feared when she learned of my past, she would run away. Why would she want to share her life with someone like me? And why would she want me to father our children – a mental health fugitive. We felt close to each other in our very different ways. We both had come through a lot. We both were dealing with a lot and probably always will. She said she felt safe with me. Not "safe-safe" – relationships are not simply safe. People have problems. Relationships have problems. There are always difficulties that tax. I don't know if it's possible for any two people not to hurt each other, and that is something I think we both knew. If a relationship is to survive, it must make room for surviving hurt. Yes, life together is painful but also more, further, a bond, caring, wanting to do well by each other, wanting to be and do better. And Rochelle was right to know that whatever hardships we went through, the kind of abuse she suffered and feared would not be part of it.

I almost felt like joking, spoiling – saying something like, "ah, but we'll create new kinds of abuse." And if that is so, wouldn't we try to catch on, correct it, use it to open new kinds of discovery? Does learning how to be together stop? I know what you're thinking. You're thinking that learning how to be with oneself doesn't stop either.

"Yes," I said. "You know me too well: Beginning never stops. The real question is does it begin?"

At this moment Philip has been with me some fourteen years, recently on and off as needed. He and Rochelle married and have three children, going through and working with what life offers. Occasional use of medication to get through rough spots, no further hospitalizations. Philip and Rochelle reached a place where they appreciate and value the humanizing challenges of everyday, always more to go.

As I sit here writing, a few "afterword" sentences come to me, and want to be communicated. They may not have been among the "great moments" of our work, but they were in small ways transformative. One is Philip talking about something Rochelle said to him fairly early in their meeting: "She said she admired my persistence in face of what I go through and that I could still be affectionate, caring, warming. She got me thinking and I began to wonder if what I went through helped make me more affectionate and caring. Just as her persisting in life through abuse and vulnerability gave her a certain kind of strength and appreciation of something better."

At another time, Philip, playing with words that mattered, stumbled on a paradoxical truth for him: "Being less made me more, and trying to be more made me less." Realities reverse and open as one lives them. "Somehow, enduring weakness brought me to this place, made me stronger."

This doesn't mean that at other times trying to be more or other isn't important. But Philip was touching an important truth for him. "My weakness brought me to a place where the little I *could* do gave me strength." A strength-in-weakness where the little good he touched (or touched him) linked with a good that permeates existence. Or if I may take a liberty, working with breakdown brought him to a tiny infinite infinitesimal point that opened life – a hard won gift.

Leda

LEDA: "I had another dream last night of dangerous water. This time, I didn't see myself in it – just the water itself, threatening to rampage. A thought came to me: "Had I already drowned?" No, definitely not. I was dreaming and I did not drown in my dream. I was twice or three times alive as the sleeper and dreamer and the absent one usually dreamt of. Was I hiding? I get the thought I was hiding behind my dream. This did not assume nightmare proportions. I didn't wake up screaming. But there was the hint of dangerous water, drowning, overpowering – or perhaps the most dangerous thing of all – being born. Being born again and again. The greatest risk. Don't you think beginning is the greatest risk? Then you are exposed, real, present. You can't get away from being. You're there, whoever you are, whatever you are. You are born."

M.E.: "You know I think beginning is the greatest gift – risk indeed! That beginning doesn't stop. The real issue is: can beginning begin?"

LEDA: "I know what you mean, but it is not so easy. I don't think you can live by formulas. Life breaks them down."

M.E.: "Yes, life is the hammer."

LEDA: "But it is our only chance. I have never recovered from childhood. I should never have been named Leda. It's all wrong. I am my father's fantasy. I was supposed to be named after my great grandmother, Lydia, but my father trapped me in a poem, a myth. He threw his mind around me like a net. How would you like to have been me, and your father reading "Leda and the Swan" throughout your childhood? By the time I was in high school, I worried that I would be in a mental hospital all my life. I am so lucky to be here talking with you, hoping for better, feeling more is possible. You should ask me why didn't I change my name? A very good question I don't have a good answer to, except when I was a child, I was proud my father valued me as a myth, a poem. Not just a little girl. A living poem. Can you imagine being a poem – your father's poem? Something you can think is good, even a blessing one moment, can be a curse the next. It was only a matter of time before I was put away again and again. For my own good. How could I ever become a person who would be here and talk with you? And you would listen – try to listen. You would hear or try to hear when you were able. I can come here and say I am a person, just me. When I say that I feel like weeping. A sorrow-anger sandwich I chew on and that eats me up. For a long time, I felt I can only be myself, try to be myself, here, but that is no longer literally true. There is more of me outside this office than there used to be, and I know it is growing – I am growing. Being here helps me grow. Helps me grow outside too, by myself, with others. I feel – and I am still testing this – am I making friends with my life? Is my life making friends with me?"

By the time this conversation – or perhaps dual monologue – took place, we were working together only seven years – more to go. Sometimes we went over the same things repeatedly. And sometimes something different entered. Meanwhile, Leda was working, exploring her own creativity, beginning to meet friends. You might say in a way the office was a kind of hospital, a place of healing or to use an old meaning, shelter. A kind of second or third skin for psychic growth. Both an escape from horror and a place to meet horror.

M.E.: "You were misused throughout your childhood."

LEDA: "A misuse that made me feel special. I was treated as special. But it was a special that blotted me out – and released me. Trapped me and gave me wings. After all – I became the swan's wings. Did the poet leave that out? Yes, Leda took on Zeus's powers, but more – she also now had wings. She could no longer be a wingless person. Perhaps I am saying we all have our special kinds of wings – but how do they become ours – my wings. Did I only have wings because of my father's wings? Or do I have wings of my own. Wings of birth?"

M.E.: "Did your father let you drop? Did he become indifferent after his pleasure?"

LEDA: "One of the scariest things was that a child of mine killed Agamemnon."

M.E.: "A child of yours became a murderess."

LEDA: "But wasn't she a part of me? Wasn't she acting out my own murderous feelings?"

M.E.: "Beautiful and murderous. What are we up against? [After a silence, I continued] We are in a danger zone. Dangerous waters. Anything can be born."

LEDA: "Yes – anything can be born."

I sat thinking about this *anything* and felt deeply touched by what therapy can offer – anything can appear in these waters, monsters, swans, beauty, death, happiness, terror, love, vast tunnels of experience, darkness and sunlight, lives lost and found, deformed and worked with – a bit akin to ancient mysteries. Stillbirths, aborted births, monster births, and births one can learn to live with – even, yes, appreciate.

M.E.: "Was there any difference between your fantasy and actual father?"

A question asked in one form or another many times. It formed itself in my mind and I shared it. I'm not sure one ever says the same thing twice – like stepping into the proverbial river. A difference in tone, nuance, ripples, waves, hopes, sense.

LEDA: "I think in my case, actual was fantasy and fantasy actual. I was swept up in my father's fantasy – I was in some way erased and enhanced by my father's fantasy. The actual man got up in the morning, worked hard, went to the bathroom, wiped crumbs from his mouth after a meal, fell asleep watching TV. But when we went to Disneyland, I almost expected to turn into one of the make-believe princesses. I half expected to be an animation. If it weren't for the actual father, I might have turned into a figment of imagination. I didn't quite put it this way before, but the actual father put the brakes on – at least some brakes. The actual father had too much weight to purely run away with himself. There were ways I survived my father's fantasy. One of them is being here talking with you. But for a long time, I never knew when I would float into space – a mind balloon. Would I ever come back? The word "brakes" makes me thing of "breaking." I don't know if one actually breaks in a breakdown or is in some ways broken all the time. But I can see that my hospital stays did bring me down to earth. Not a very pleasant way to be brought down. Brought back. It was awful in its own ways. But it was something undeniably happening to me, not a fantasy. It was a reality. I remember the moment it came to me that I was someone I had to take care of, that needed care. And that the care I received growing up brought me to a point where I could begin to glimpse the care I needed. It brought me to breakdown. It took time, but I finally saw I could not take care of myself and had a lot of learning to do. I think therapy is a place of learning, a school I never had, school about feelings. A place to let some ice melt. You like using the term "psychic gymnasium" for therapy, a place you exercise capacities a little differently. Discover ways of working with yourself. Now I know all of life is a gym, a school, if one gets the feel of how to tap into it and not be washed away, destroyed."

M.E.: "The dangerous waters."

LEDA: "Dangerous, life-giving waters. Now I associate the word breakdown with beginning: breakdown-beginning. A reality one learns to work with."

M.E.: "All life long."

After sitting a while, my mind goes back to dream waters and r-words: ravished, ravaged, rampage. I find myself saying them out loud, and Leda replies with her own r-word.

LEDA: "Raped by father's mind all through childhood, fantasy father feathers – rape that never stops, a soft rape. Maybe a caring rape as well – a kind of father caring mixed in. I was his little girl, his princess. Daddy's girl. Mental abuse can be very subtle, a wind lifting one into the air. Coming down hard in hospitals. One needs help – really needs help."

M.E. "And your mother? Where did she come in?"

LEDA: "You're thinking, why didn't she save me from my father? She couldn't save herself. I get the idea that therapy tries to help me save me from myself – helps me grow tools to try to live a little better."

M.E.: "Your remark makes me think of a person I learned a lot from who said therapy helps introduce the patient to herself. But here it is more, learning a little better to save one from oneself."

We sit quietly for some time, letting the session sink in more. An awful thought begins to come to me. Should I say it or wait to see where it goes? It tumbles out in all its awfulness:

M.E.: "I'm wondering if self-destruction can be a way of cleaning oneself out, getting rid of fantasies that bind you, getting rid of being your father's fantasy."

LEDA: "I think I see what you're saying. Cleaning myself out of things that suffocate by destroying myself – destroying what enables the invasion to bind."

M.E.: "Some people destroy self, aspects of self, thoughts, feelings, body . . ."

LEDA: "Zeroing oneself as way to begin to be."

We didn't meet for several weeks, owing to a business trip Leda took. When she came back, she was eager to talk about a dream she had about her mother.

LEDA: "She was sitting in a small room she made for herself, her sewing room. She did some sewing by hand, some with a machine. An old black machine she would bend over with a bright light. She could vary the light to see different shadings. In my dream, she looked like she did in real life, except her lips seemed more determined and her fingers and hands more persistent. She seemed somehow stronger, as if she could bend over her work longer without feeling much pain. She had more lasting power. Her eyes lit up when I looked at them – this was a strange thing because I was not in the dream. It was a solo for her – she and her sewing. The material looked like a soft maroon. But when I, as the dreamer, looked at her eyes, they lit up in the dream. It was like a thin veil between me, the dreamer, and she, the dreamt, and my looking at her could affect her expression. I am surprised by my dream and have so much to talk about. I don't know if I can find it all. I am seeing myself as a baby with my mother in her own world and yet affect her, her eyes glow when I look at them. She is busy with her own tasks. She was always busy with something, housework, office work. Maybe also busy with me, attending to diapers, attending to feeding. I have a feeling I could not affect her, but in the dream, I can affect her in some way. I can turn a light in her on. When I say that a light in me goes off and on. When I try to imagine it the off-on goes faster, slower, faster, slower. I'm wondering what you are thinking – seeing?"

M.E.: "I'm wondering about rhythms in the psyche, rhythms of being. Wondering if the baby or child lives them without knowing what they are. They can be pretty baffling, turning on and off with each other and ourselves. It is a wonderful description you are giving."

LEDA: "We can be there and not there at the same time or in different ways. It's not so surprising. We vanish for a time when sleeping and come back again. Why shouldn't there be ways we disappear and return when awake?"

M.E.: "You spoke of a thin veil between states."

LEDA: "Thank God for the veil. I think when the veil disappeared, I had to be hospitalized. The veil keeps me out of hospital."

M.E.: "Let's you experience things and explore them at the same time."

LEDA: "There are good ways to have distance or the impact is too much, too final. You get caught in a scream. Here we can try to stay in contact and go on living. That is one of the most amazing things our work has helped me with: surviving contact with myself."

We were quiet for a while. To me, the quiet felt like a prayer, but I am aware that is something I often feel. Perhaps for her it was a time to breathe, a moment of appreciation. I didn't have time to ask, as Leda began talking about something that concerned her.

LEDA: "I really need to say more about my mother in the dream. It was so unusual to picture her as so quiet, still, absorbed. As if she was having a good moment of aloneness. Oddly, my seeing her alone did not make me feel more alone. It made me feel more present in a still, quiet way. When I think of the persistence, determination, and strength I saw in the dream, I wonder if I am not using her to convey something in me that has come through so much, and continues coming through. It's been such a struggle. But here we are, continuing. My life keeps living and living me. And I keep living my life. Who would have thought this possible? There were no bad voices in the dream. No voices demanding I do something horrible, no attacks. This in itself is amazing, my dream mother in a quiet moment with no bad voices. Let me apply this to myself – a quiet moment with myself that feels good. Not battling bad presences. Time off. I'm smiling. I'm aware that Mom did not stand up to my father and create a better balance. But my dream mother is getting better and I am too. I know it will always be hard. Being a person is not easy. I suspect there are strengths and awfulness from both parents that invaded and supported me, and strengths and awfulness in my own relation to myself. Somehow, I survived being crushed and now I'm growing. Growing is another kind of difficulty filled with difficulties worth a try."

What a blessing, to have moments free of bad voices attacking, pressures of internal commands one dare not fulfil. I doubt bad voices ever completely vanish, but they can lessen, take up a little less room, and with further work become tendencies one can partly explore. When I heard Leda speak of past and present difficulties and difficulties to come, I thought of some of Sigmund Freud's last words on a recording he made near the end of his life. He was speaking about psychoanalysis and the psychoanalytic movement. The words I am thinking of: "And the struggle is not yet over." A week later, she found herself speaking about a war between mothers.

LEDA: "Since my recent mother dream, I've been feeling a struggle between two mothers in me. One that is slowly getting better, while another remains the same or is getting worse. As though the better one mother gets, the worse the other becomes. One becomes more generous, the other more tyrannical. One supports, one tears down."

M.E.: "It sounds like the negative mother won't leave go as a more positive one gets born and grows."

LEDA: "Yes, that's what I'm feeling."

M.E.: "I'm wondering if you are glimpsing two states or tendencies that are mixed or fused and now they are separating out as you grow more capable of sustaining what's in you."

LEDA: "And moments that are neither one nor the other."

M.E.: "Exactly. More freedom to feel yourself in a fuller way, not just tied by one or the other."

A week later, Leda came in fearing all the good and strength were falling away. The self-sustaining mother in her dream collapsed into the real-life mother who had to be hospitalized when Leda was 2 and again when she was 5. We talked much about her mother's breakdowns, the fear she had that there was no footing in life. Weak mother, angry mother, crying mother. The mind can open like a hole and vanish into itself any moment – or worse, horrible beings can appear relentless in their attacks.

LEDA: "There is something different about this collapse. I have a lot of thoughts about it. My collapse tied to my mother's collapse. If she goes, I go. But she is still alive living her life, and so am I. We are survivors – and more. At least I feel something more now – I feel like a student of life. I am not sure what I'm learning, but I'm learning."

M.E.: "I feel I hear you saying that in your life good survives bad and you survive both."

LEDA: "Good is real beyond struggle. There is something more than its life-and-death struggle with the bad. This may be crazy, but I'm feeling good is good in itself and bad feeds off it. I think this is what I was reaching for in my breakdowns: good in itself, for its own sake, because it is. It can't be defined by fight, although fight is part of it. It has deeper roots in life itself. I'm beginning to see good and bad can exist as different moments, not just against each other. When I feel that I can breathe. Breathing in and out is not against each other. They are part of breathing, like crying and laughing are part of living. Is it true or am I kidding myself – there is more to life than its struggle with death?"

Conclusion

Alma, Philip, Leda – three different journeys through depths of breakdown, now hospital free. So much of our work had to do with moment to moment impact, nuances of states shifting, reversals and rhythms of closing-opening, staying with the call of experience. A perennial struggle is whether good can survive bad, and what would that look like. Is life worth living – and how? Is it possible for the human psyche to build tolerance for itself and in what ways? How much of oneself can one take? In various ways, we touched possibilities of growth.

Work with psychosis has been an important thread in my work from the beginning. My first book, *The Psychotic Core* (1986), focused on basic dynamics of areas of psychosis, and later work (e.g., 2004, 2009, 2011, 2019) opened further possibilities. We like to joke that we are mad and life is crazy, and that can lighten some moments. But in truth, there is much we must keep learning to work with, some taxing what we are capable of and perhaps even stimulating further evolution of capacities, learning to be better partners with ourselves. A work, after all these thousands of years, we are still beginning. That, perhaps, is one of our greatest learnings of all: learning to begin – a learning that is ever in question but does not stop calling.

References

Bion, W. R. (1970). *Attention and interpretation*. London: Routledge.

Eigen, M. (1986/2018). *The psychotic core*. London: Routledge.

Eigen, M. (2002). A basic rhythm. *Psychoanalytic Review*, *88*, 455–481.

Eigen, M. (2004). *The sensitive self*. Middletown, CT: Wesleyan University Press.

Eigen, M. (2005). *Emotional storm*. Middletown, CT: Wesleyan University Press.

Eigen, M. (2009/2018). *Flames from the unconscious: Trauma, madness and faith*. London: Routledge.

Eigen, M. (2011/2018). *Contact with the depths*. London: Routledge.

Eigen, M. (2019). *Dialogues with Michael eigen: Psyche singing*. London: Routledge.

Winnicott, D. W. (1965/1992). The psychology of madness. In C. Winnicott, R. Shepherd, & M. Davis (Eds.), *Psychoanalytic explorations* (pp. 119–130). Cambridge, MA: Harvard University Press.

Index

For Product Safety Concerns and Information please contact our EU
representative GPSR@taylorandfrancis.com
Taylor & Francis Verlag GmbH, Kaufingerstraße 24, 80331 München, Germany

www.ingramcontent.com/pod-product-compliance
Lightning Source LLC
Chambersburg PA
CBHW070336270326
41926CB00017B/3887